INFECTION CONTROL MANUAL FOR HEALTHCARE PROFESSIONALS

Liz Shipsey-Eldridge
Janet Kerswell Unnasch

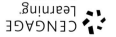

CENGAGE Learning

Infection Control Manual for Healthcare Professionals
1st Edition
Liz Shipsey-Eldridge
Janet Kerswell Unnasch

Publishing manager: Dorothy Chiu
Associate publishing editor: Chee Ng
Developmental editor: Tharaka Richards
Project editors: Michaela Skelly & Amelia Fellows
Art direction: Danielle Maccarone
Cover designer: Emilie Pfitzner (Everyday Ambition)
Text designer: Danielle Maccarone
Editor: Julie Wicks
Proofreader: Jill Pope
Indexer: Julie King
Permissions/Photo researcher: QZA Media
Cover: iStockphoto/posterior
Typeset by MPS Limited

Any URLs contained in this publication were checked for currency during the production process. Note, however, that the publisher cannot vouch for the ongoing currency of URLs.

This first edition published in 2016

National Library of Australia Cataloguing-in-Publication Data

Creator: Shipsey-Eldridge, Liz, author.
Title: *Infection Control Manual for Healthcare Professionals* /
Liz Shipsey-Eldridge, Janet Kerswell Unnasch.
ISBN: 9780170261609 (paperback)
Subjects: Communicable diseases--Nursing--Study and teaching--Australia.
Communicable diseases--Prevention--Study and teaching--Australia.
Infection--Study and teaching--Australia.
Nursing--Study and teaching--Australia.
Other Creators/Contributors: Kerswell Unnasch, Janet, author.
Dewey Number: 616.9071094

Cengage Learning Australia
Level 7, 80 Dorcas Street
South Melbourne, Victoria Australia 3205

Cengage Learning New Zealand
Unit 4B Rosedale Office Park
331 Rosedale Road, Albany, North Shore 0632, NZ

For learning solutions, visit **cengage.com.au**

Printed in China by 1010 Printing International Limited.
1 2 3 4 5 6 7 19 18 17 16 15

BRIEF CONTENTS

CONTENTS

PREFACE

Healthcare workers and their clients are continually exposed to microorganisms due to the nature of the clinical environment. Healthcare associated infections (HAIs) have become an increasingly burgeoning problem for all healthcare settings. According to the National Health and Medical Research Council (NHMRC) (2010), HAIs account for approximately 200000 infections per year in the Australian acute care setting alone.

HAIs are the single most common problem experienced by clients, exclusive of the reason for hospitalisation in most healthcare settings. These complications are clearly demonstrated by:

- increased duration of illness
- longer recovery times
- economic losses to the client (e g lost work time)
- higher incidence of antibiotic prescribing
- heightened costs to the facility
- greater workload for healthcare workers
- significant mortality rates that can be attributed to HAIs.

It is critical to note that many of these HAIs are actually preventable and healthcare workers are pivotal in both transmission and reduction of infections.

Infection Control Manual for Healthcare Professionals aims to educate students and staff working in the healthcare setting, by providing valuable underpinning knowledge and an insight into the skills required to reduce infection transmission based on principles of prevention and control.

The manual has been designed to have a dual role in relation to education and training. The knowledge and skills contained within each chapter have been directly drawn from the government's vocational education training website, http://www.training.gov.au. It ensures that all content has been mapped to the unit of competency *comply with infection control policies and procedures* and includes mapping to the *essential skills and knowledge* alongside all *elements and performance criteria*.

The primary purpose of this text is to provide healthcare students with a comprehensive understanding of infection control. It is written in an informative and user-friendly style so that students can acquire the skills and knowledge base for practical application. As the text has been mapped against the Infection control competency, it serves as a perfect learning tool to accompany the assessment items.

In addition, it is a useful educational resource in almost any clinical setting. For example, the appendices, workplace orientation and infectious outbreak management sections can be used as part of a formalised orientation for new staff or as an annual update for existing staff. Alternatively, sections such as a viral outbreak in a facility may be utilised in times of crisis thus acting as a quick and straightforward guide to the management of most pandemics commonly experienced in Australia's varying healthcare settings.

LANGUAGE AND TERMINOLOGY

As this textbook has a full chapter on health issues pertaining to Aboriginal and Torres Straits Islander peoples, we have sought to use inclusive, appropriate and non-discriminatory terminology throughout. For this purpose we have, with Aunty Kerrie Doyle's advice, closely followed the published guidelines provided by NSW Health in *Communicating Positively: A Guide to Appropriate Aboriginal Terminology.*

ABOUT THE AUTHORS

Liz Shipsey-Eldridge, RN, BN, Masters of Public Health (Health promotion), Cert IV in TAE, Grad Dip Higher Ed, is a senior clinical nurse and educator in aged care. She has previously taught both the Diploma of Nursing (Enrolled – Division 2) and the Certificate III in Aged Care for over seven years. She has also worked in adolescent mental health in London, and in community-based nursing. She has extensive experience in palliative care and is currently conducting an intense palliative care education program in her workplace. Liz is passionate about excellence in patient care in all facets of nursing. She is a self-professed 'born teacher' and endeavours to do so in any role she undertakes. She has returned to work in industry at this time.

The authors and Cengage Learning extend special thanks to Aunty Kerrie Doyle, Associate Professor (Indigenous Health) from RMIT University, for contributing to *Chapter 5: Cultural considerations in Australian healthcare* and for her generous guidance and advice regarding cultural diversity in Australian healthcare settings.

Janet Kerswell Unnasch, RN, Grad Dip Mental Health (Distinction), Cert IV in TAE, is a guest lecturer for the Institute of Continuing and TESOL Education University of Queensland (ICTE–UQ). She has taught the Diploma of Nursing (Enrolled – Division 2) for the past eight years across on campus, online and distance education settings. She has a passion for 'reaching' students via the written word. Janet is committed to improving the patients' lived experience of palliative and end-of-life care as well as increasing the general public's understanding of mental health conditions and actively reducing stigma experienced by consumers. Janet has also returned to work in industry at this time.

ACKNOWLEDGEMENTS

This book would not have been possible without the support of our family and colleagues. Thanks must also go to our external reviewers who gave valuable feedback and advice on each of the chapters in order to improve the relevance of the text in Australia and New Zealand. The team at Cengage have been incredible and a pleasure to work with – a special thank you to Chee Ng (publishing editor), Tharaha Richards (development editor), Michaela Skelly (project editor) and Julie Wicks (editor), who have been incredibly patient and supportive beyond expectation.

From Liz: I could not have done this without the support of my family including my mum Dorelle, my sister Kath, my brother Brett and daughter Charlotte who tolerated all the weekends I have spent on this away from them! A very special mention to my husband, Tim Shipsey, who passed away in January 2015, part way through the development process. Tim, I thank you for your inspiration and the amazing gift you gave me in our daughter, Charlotte Christina Ellen Shipsey.

From Janet: I would like to thank my long-suffering husband, Des, for his incredible support during this writing process. No request made of him was too big or too small. He lead a band of equally diligent helpers who supplied our frequent calls for food, cool drinks and most importantly coffee! To my daughters Serena and Chloe, and their friends Bill, Jarrod and Malachi, please accept our thanks for your tireless work in running back and forward to the kitchen to deliver our demands! Whether this effort was given through love or fear we may never know; however, it was greatly appreciated by both Liz and me. To my son Drew, my daughter Elise and my brother David, please accept my thanks for your encouragement, which was delivered in many obscure ways. To my cousin Melinda, who threw a lifeline to both Liz and me when we needed it most … you are a legend! Finally, to my parents Bill, Mavis and Joy, thank you for always believing in me.

Liz Shipsey-Eldridge and Janet Kerswell Unnasch

Cengage Learning would like to thank the following lecturers who provided feedback on the plans for this text in the early stages of its development or reviewed draft chapters, as well as those who provided anonymous feedback:

Pamela Cronin – TAFE Qld Brisbane
Christine Baker – Swinburne University of Technology
Gale Cowled – TAFE NSW Riverina Institute
Anne Moates – Chisholm Institute of TAFE
Carol Barbeler – Central Gippsland Institute of TAFE
Lindsay Bava – Kangan Institute of TAFE
Loretta Alexander – North Coast Institute of TAFE
Sister Jennifer Farrell – University of Notre Dame
Erin Cable – Goldfields Institute of Technology
Maree Le Fevre – Metropolitan South Institute of TAFE
Beth Rutherford – Sydney Institute of TAFE

Guide to the text

As you read this text you will find a number of features in every chapter to enhance your study of infection control.

EXAMPLE

Example boxes illustrate key concepts throughout the text.

EXAMPLE

Clinical examples of infection from different modes of transmission and varying reservoirs

- A person with a respiratory infection such as *tuberculosis* broadcasts infectious *droplets* through coughing and sneezing.
- Surgical wounds can easily become infected if normal flora from the skin (e.g. *Staphlococcus epidermis*) enters the compromised site via *direct contact*.
- There have been several cases of humans contracting

CASE STUDY

Case studies showcase real-life scenarios, to make your learning more meaningful.

CASE STUDY

Minimising waste

A new national waste management initiative has been implemented across a variety of industries, including healthcare. Anglicare (a community-based nursing service) in South Australia has joined the campaign to eliminate the production of industry-created waste. The program is called *Zero Waste*.

Anglicare has managed to divert general and clinical waste from landfill sites. In a small timeframe (approximately six weeks) the initiative has increased re-direction and

Tip boxes emphasise the key clinical concepts you will need to consider.

TIP BOX

Treating worm infestations
It is very important that the whole family be treated at the same time as the infected child, alongside any bedding and clothing that may have been affected.

Test your understanding of important concepts with the **activities** throughout each chapter.

ACTIVITY

Reading a pathology report
Use the pathology report in Figure 6.2 and answer the following questions.
1   What type of specimen does this pathology report provide results for?
2   From which part of the body was the specimen collected?
3   Name the antibiotic the infective organism is resistant to.
4   Name the antibiotics the infective organism is sensitive to.
5   Name the infective organism.

END OF CHAPTER FEATURES

At the end of the chapter you will find:

- a summary of key points
- review questions.

SUMMARY

- Organisational policies and procedures form the fundamental basis for effective infection control practices.
- Healthcare organisations are obliged to provide comprehensive policies and procedures that are easily accessible to staff.
- Healthcare workers are obliged to accurately implement policies and procedures and acknowledge the link they have to current legislation.
- It is imperative that healthcare workers are acutely aware of circumstances requiring the implementation of specific policies and procedures.

- Infection control policies and procedures, once accessed and understood, must be acted upon.
- Interventions that require prompt application of infection control policies and procedures must be accompanied by an evaluation process.
- It is crucial to acknowledge that these actions contribute to the overall quality improvement in infection control and healthcare practices.

REVIEW QUESTIONS

1 Discuss the importance and goal of staff immunisation policies.
2 Which document would you refer to in order to ascertain your facility's approved method for inserting an indwelling urinary catheter? Where would you expect to find this information?

3 Discuss your understanding of the quality improvement process and your associated role.
4 Discuss the role of the public health unit.
5 A new health worker approaches you for direction regarding emptying a urinary catheter bag. Discuss your response.

At the end of the book you will find:

- appendices covering Australian, State and Territory legislative requirements for infection control, and summaries of safe infection control practices, including outbreak management procedures
- a glossary of key terms from throughout the text.

APPENDIX A: AUSTRALIAN, STATE AND TERRITORY LEGISLATIVE REQUIREMENTS

Overarching Commonwealth laws, also referred to as Acts, detail health and safety concepts, among others, that are directly related to infection control and safe practise. Regulations are a set of mandatory requirements that comply with an Act. Every State and Territory of Australia has its own interpretation of the Act, and thus its own Regulations. The local health and safety authority then administers these regulations, hence why the laws vary across the country.

The following table lists the relevant legislation and standards in Australia, inclusive of States and Territories, that pertain to infection control within the healthcare environment.

	Standards and legislation	Topics covered
Australia	**Work Health and Safety Act 2011**	
ACT	Work Health and Safety Regulation 2011 SL2011-36 Republication number 17, effective from 21 May 2015 Administered by Work Safe Australian Capital Territory (www.worksafe.act.gov.au)	• Workplace health and safety • Standard and transmission-based precautions, including the use of PPE
QLD	Work Health and Safety Regulation 2011 Effective from 24 October 2014 Administered by Workplace Health and Safety Queensland (https://www.worksafe.qld.gov.au/)	• Safe handling and disposal of sharps
NSW	Work Health and Safety Reg Effective from 4 June 2015 Administered by the Work-Cove	
TAS	Work Health and Safety Reg Administered by Workplace Sta	
SA	Work Health and Safety Reg Administered by SafeWork SA	

GLOSSARY

access relates to how easy or difficult it is for a person to obtain healthcare services and/or advice

aerobic an organism that must have oxygen in order to survive and grow

airborne carried through the air

airborne precautions guidelines used for patients who are known to be infected and have the possibility of infection transmission via the airborne route

alcohol-based hand rub (ABHR) alcohol-based preparation that is rubbed onto hands with the view of reducing microorganisms and does not require the use of running water as it evaporates

allied health worker (AHW) physiotherapists, occupational therapists, speech pathologists, social workers, podiatrists and their assistants

amoebae a single-celled protozoa that utilises pseudopods to move (eukaryotic organism)

anaerobic an organism that must not have oxygen in order to survive and grow

antibiotic a group of medications that are often used to treat bacterial infections

antibodies a protein produced by the body in response to infection; they are found in the blood and other body fluids; the immunoglobulins are produced by lymphocytes in response to bacteria, viruses and other infections

assistant in nursing (AIN) a worker who has undertaken Certificate III level studies in an area of healthcare, such as aged care; some healthcare providers no longer offer assistant-in-nursing positions, preferring to employ people as personal care workers

asymptomatic without symptoms

bacteria a microorganism that may be capable of causing disease (prokaryotic organism)

bacterial spores see endospores

bloodborne viruses (BBVs) viruses that are present in a person's blood and can be transmitted through direct contact with the infected person's blood or bodily fluids; they include HIV, hepatitis B and hepatitis C

bronchoscope an instrument used to examine the bronchus, the large airways of the lungs

candidiasis an overgrowth of *Candida albicans* causing a fungal condition

carrier a person who carries a pathogen with or without symptoms of disease

central line an intravenous line or catheter that is inserted into a large vein (such as the superior vena cava) typically in the neck, to rest near the heart

chemotherapeutic the effect of chemicals that have a toxic effect on microorganisms causing disease or that selectively destroy tumour tissues

chemotherapy refers to the use of any drug to treat disease; however, it is usually used to describe drug therapy used to treat cancer

125

Guide to the online resources

FOR THE INSTRUCTOR

Cengage Learning is pleased to provide you with a selection of resources that will help you prepare your lectures and assessments. These teaching tools are accessible via http://login.cengage.com.

INSTRUCTOR'S MANUAL
The instructor's manual includes:
- suggested responses for in-chapter activities and case studies, and end-of-chapter review questions
- weblinks.

TEST BANK
A test bank of questions, covering the core unit of competency as well as the learning objectives and key topics, has been prepared for your use. The questions are available in Word file format and can be uploaded directly into your Learning Management System or customised to meet your students' learning requirements.

POWERPOINT™ PRESENTATIONS
Use the chapter-by-chapter PowerPoint slides to enhance your lecture presentations and to reinforce the key principles of your subject, or for student handouts.

ARTWORK FROM THE TEXT
Add the digital files of graphs, pictures and flowcharts into your course management system, use them within student handouts or copy them into lecture presentations.

DETAILED MAPPING GRID
A detailed competency mapping grid shows you how the core unit of competency *Comply with infection control policies and procedures* is covered in this book.

LESSON PLANS
The lesson plans provide guidance for instructors, helping them plan, deliver and assess students against the learning objectives and performance criteria.

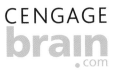

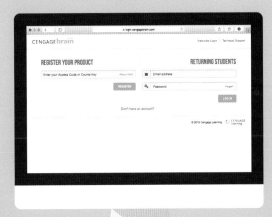

Visit the Infection Control Manual for Healthcare Professionals companion website. You'll find:

- revision quizzes
- internet research activities
- and more tools to help you excel in your studies.

1. BASIC MICROBIOLOGY AND INFECTIOUS DISEASES

LEARNING OBJECTIVES

At the end of this chapter, you will be able to:

- explain the concepts of basic microbiology
- describe bacteria and fungi
- identify viruses, including bacteria and spores, fungi, viruses, protozoa and helminths
- describe resident and transient flora.

Introduction

The first chapter focuses on basic microbiology concepts to lay the foundation for further learning. This chapter will explore the common types of microorganisms relevant to healthcare settings. It will also outline the significance and meaning of both resident and transient flora. The chapter will then focus on how these factors interrelate with common **infections** and **diseases**, alongside a brief explanation of associated treatments. Last, this chapter will discuss certain aspects of infectious agents and pathogens and the implications these can have in a healthcare setting. This final segment will also consider the role of opportunistic organisms and the virulent role they play in healthcare.

Basic microbiology concepts

Microbiology is the study of what is commonly referred to as germs, known as **microorganisms** in the healthcare setting. These microorganisms include terms that the reader may already be familiar with, such as **bacteria**, **fungi** and **viruses**. It is important to note that 'micro', meaning small, indicates that microorganisms cannot be seen with the naked eye.

Microorganisms are broken into two distinct groups, **eukaryotic** and **prokaryotic**, and are differentiated on the basis of structure and function. A eukaryotic microorganism is defined as one that has at least one cell, including a nucleus, and other structures called organelles required for efficient functioning. These types of cells are larger and more complex than their counterparts, the prokaryotic-based microorganisms.

Conversely, the prokaryotic cell is far simpler and less structured, containing only one single cell but enclosed by a cell wall. Unlike the eukaryotic cell, it does not contain other structures such as organelles for higher level functioning.

Bacteria

All bacteria meet the benchmarks for classification as prokaryotic microorganisms. Bacteria (prokaryotic-based cells) are one of the most commonly known but potentially infectious microorganisms. They are quite simple in structure (refer to **Figure 1.1**) as they are single-celled organisms; however, they can survive either as independent entities or dependent on another **organism**.

FIGURE 1.1 Pneumococcal disease is a bacterial infection caused by the *Streptococcus pneumoniae* (*S. pneumoniae*), often referred to as pneumococcus

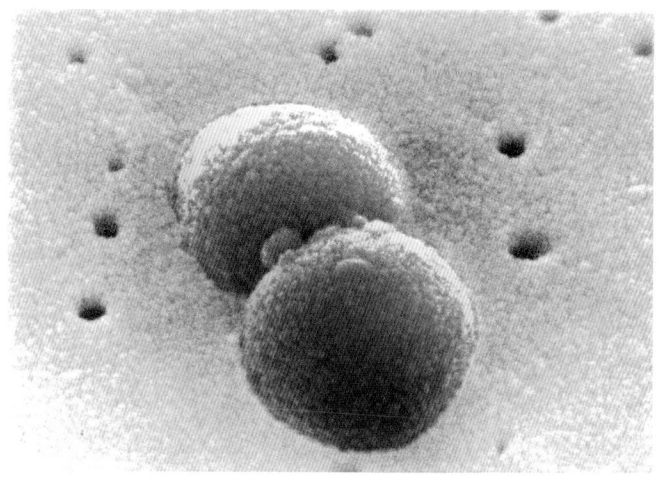

Source: BSIP/UIG Via Getty Images

Bacteria: Basic facts

A bacterium (singular) is a unicellular prokaryotic microorganism that usually multiplies by cell division; it has a cell wall that provides a constancy of form; it may be **aerobic** or **anaerobic**; motile or non-motile; free-living, saprophytic, parasitic or pathogenic.

Bacteria: Naming structure

Bacteria usually have at least two names, sometimes three. The first name is the **genus** (general classification group) and the second is the type of **species**; the third name may indicate a particular **strain**. For example,

- Genus = Escherichia
- Species = coli
- Strain = O157
- Bacteria name = *Escherichia coli* O157
  The wording will often be abbreviated; for example, *E. coli*.

Bacteria: Morphology

Morphology simply means the shape of something, and all bacteria are classified in accordance with their shape. **Table 1.1** below outlines the common bacterial names that reflect the bacteria's shape.

Bacteria: Classification

Bacteria are classified in accordance with their different features and shapes. The most significant test to establish the classification of bacteria is by using the **Gram** staining technique.

TABLE 1.1 Morphology of bacteria

Morphology title	Description	Picture
Coccus	Coccus stems from the word *kokkos* (meaning *berry*) and are oval shaped in appearance. Common types of coccus include diplococci (meaning *double* or *in pairs*), staphylococci (meaning *in clusters*) and streptococci (meaning *in chains*).	 Source: BSIP SA/Alamy
Bacillus	A rod-shaped bacteria.	 Source: Eraxion/iStockphoto
Coccobacillus	Coccobacilli are a combination of the two types of bacteria above and their shape is a combination of a rod and an oval.	 Source: Dennis Kunkel Microscopy, Inc./Visuals Unlimited/Corbis

Morphology title	Description	Picture
Spirillum	Spirillum are firm and inflexible in nature but are spiral in appearance.	 Source: Michael Abbey/Getty Images
Spirochetes	Spirochetes stems from the words *speira* (*coil*) and *chaite* (*hair-like*). They appear as thin flexible coils.	 Source: Juergen Berger/Science Photo Library

Using the Gram staining technique

Hans Christian Gram introduced the staining system in 1884 as a method of identifying the different types of bacteria. This is still the benchmark today, used to distinguish bacteria into two main groups: **Gram positive** (+) and **Gram negative** (−). The process involves staining bacteria with different types of substances such as iodine, purple dye, alcohol decolourisation and safranin.

The bacteria that retain the dye colour have robust cell walls and are considered to be the Gram positive types of bacteria, while those that lose the pigment have permeable cell walls and cannot contain the dye as effectively and are therefore classified as Gram negative bacteria.

Acid-fast bacteria

The next type of bacterial classification is the acid-fast bacteria, with the genus name of *Mycobacterium*. It is a slightly different type of staining test but is able to distinguish this type of bacteria from both the Gram positive and Gram negative classifications. Examples include *Mycobacterium tuberculosis* (tuberculosis) and *Mycobacterium leprae* (leprosy).

Aerobic and anaerobic bacteria

This concept basically refers to whether the bacteria require oxygen to survive and grow. Aerobic bacteria need oxygen while anaerobic bacteria do not. However, there are some bacteria that have managed to mutate and adapt to differing environments despite their original requirements. Many of these bacteria are found in the human gut.

Bacterial spores

Spores are single-celled entities capable of reproductive functions. Some bacteria are able to produce **endospores** within the primary cell. They are generally known to be resistant to normal cleansing techniques such as boiling, heating and disinfecting.

The significance of spores in the healthcare setting is reflected in **sterilisation** efficiency. The presence or absence of spores after sterilisation has occurred will indicate whether they have been eradicated or not.

The following information about bacterial symptoms, **transmission**, susceptibility, diagnosis and treatment is based on a particular strain called methicillin-resistant *Staphylococcus aureus* (MRSA).

Example of a bacterial infection: MRSA

While there are many different types of bacteria that concern the healthcare professional, we will focus on one of the most clinically significant types: *Staphylococcus aureus*. It is actually a naturally occurring (that is, part of the **normal flora**) bacteria found on many people in our population and tends to thrive best in locations such as the skin, nose, arm pits and groin. As the name suggests, it is a vigorous bacteria that can overcome the strength of methicillin-based **antibiotics** as well as some other antibiotics.

There are two strains of Staphylococcus aureus that are of particular concern to the **healthcare worker (HCW)** as they both have the ability to debilitate clients. The first strain of staph is called **methicillin-resistant** *Staphylococcus aureus* (MRSA) (commonly referred to as **staph**) and is one of the most well-known bacteria, especially in a clinical setting (see **Figure 1.2**). The second type is found outside most clinical settings and is more prevalent in the community. It is called non-multiresistant MRSA (nmMRSA) and, while it may sound less hazardous than MRSA, it potentially can be more problematic because it can easily affect healthy people who have limited, if any, risk factors for infection.

MRSA symptoms

As MRSA commonly occurs on the skin, it is not surprising that many people will present with skin infections that are characterised by:

- swelling
- pain

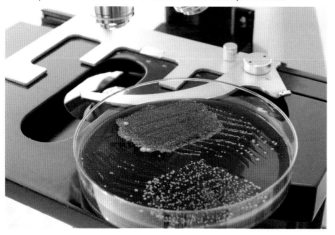

Source: Zaharia Bogdan Rares/Shutterstock

- redness
- heat
- a wound of some kind, such as an abscess.

TIP BOX

Survival of MRSA

MRSA is so stubborn that it can even stick to plastic and survive!

If the immune system is not compromised and therefore performing well, symptoms may be mild and localised to that particular area of skin. However, it is possible that the bacteria can spread throughout the whole body and therefore is classified as a **systemic infection**. When a systemic infection occurs, the whole body is usually affected and not just the original site of infection. Symptoms can include:

- fever
- shaking
- fatigue
- shortness of breath
- rigors (uncontrollable shakes).

This needs immediate medical attention, possibly hospital admission, and commencement of antibiotic therapy as it is potentially life-threatening.

MRSA transmission

MRSA is usually transmitted via direct contact with a person who is either infected with the bacteria or, at the very least, carries it on their skin or other areas already identified as high-risk sites.

Commonly, the transmission occurs through close skin contact and surfaces that are frequently touched. Although this is a problem in the clinical setting, it is more probable when ineffective and infrequent handwashing principles are not strictly applied.

It is not uncommon for clients with a known case of MRSA to be placed in a single room (**isolation**) and staff will take extra measures (**transmission-based precautions**) to prevent the spread by using more specialised medical aids such as personal protective equipment (PPE), which will be discussed in detail in Chapter 4.

MRSA susceptibility

Although anyone can become infected with MRSA, it is more common in people with a heightened susceptibility. These people include but are not limited to:

- the elderly
- the young
- those with compromised immune systems
- those with wounds
- those with intravenous drips
- those with more than one medical condition, especially diabetics
- those who are frequently in highly or overpopulated areas such as healthcare facilities and child care centres.

MRSA diagnosis

If MRSA infection is suspected, a swab (or small scraping) of the affected area needs to be taken and sent to a pathology laboratory for testing (as shown in **Figure 1.3**). This will then establish exactly what microorganism is present in that area and which antibiotics are best suited to treat it.

MRSA treatment

Dependent on the site of infection, treatment could involve procedures such as draining of an abscess or skin lesion.

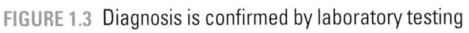

FIGURE 1.3 Diagnosis is confirmed by laboratory testing

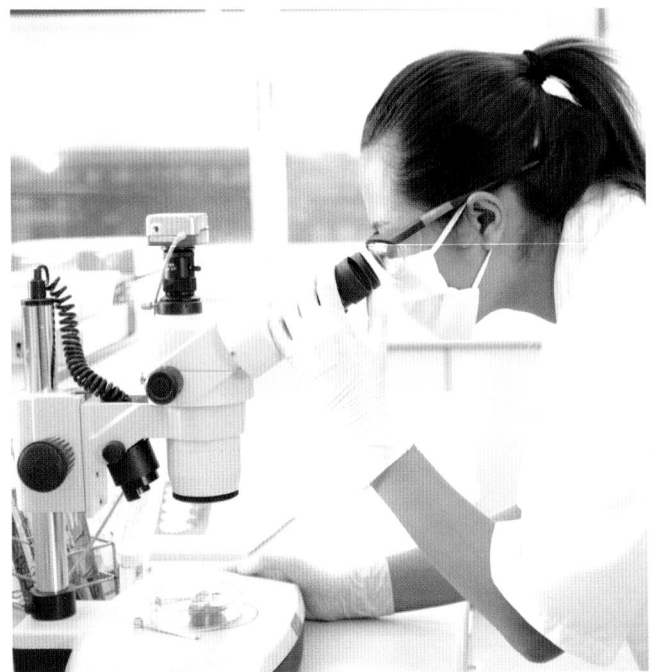

Source: SOMKKU/Shutterstock

Antibiotics (**Figure 1.4**) are usually prescribed in accordance with the pathology results. It is important to encourage clients to complete the set course of antibiotics even once signs and symptoms of the infection have eased. Recurrence of the underlying infection is quite common if the course of antibiotics is not completed. Incomplete courses can also encourage a level of antibiotic resistance to the MRSA.

EXAMPLE

Impetigo, commonly known as school sores

The summary below provides an example of a well-known bacterial infection and associated treatments.

* School sores, otherwise known as *impetigo*, is a common but highly contagious bacterial infection of the skin.
* The causative bacteria are either *Staphylococcus aureus* or *Streptococcal pyogenes* (strep), which gain entry to the body via a small cut, bite or even a break in the skin from eczema.
* Typically, blisters form which can vary in size depending on which bacteria is present.
* Staph infections tend to produce large fluid-filled blisters.
* Strep infections tend to be much smaller.
* Blisters should be covered with a clean or sterile dressing to reduce the risk of transmission to others and avoid contracting a secondary bacterial infection.
* Children are usually kept away from school until the blisters have dried out and the risk of transmission is lowered.
* The usual course of treatment includes oral antibiotics and also antibiotic cream for application to blisters.

FIGURE 1.4 Antibiotics are prescribed to treat bacterial infections

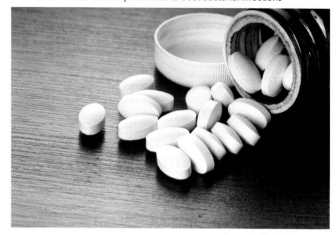

Source: Ahuli Labutin/Shutterstock

Fungi

Fungi, as shown in **Figure 1.5**, are varying clusters of eukaryotic organisms that survive on decomposing organic matter. They are usually single celled and present quite differently to other microorganisms. Fungi are also used to produce medications to help treat various conditions.

FIGURE 1.5 Fungi

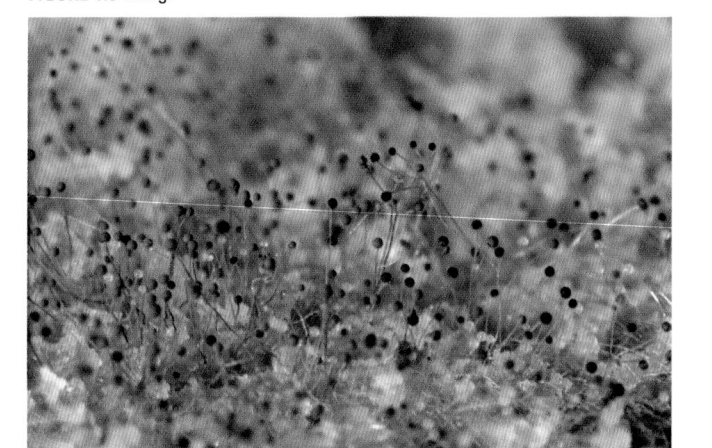

Source: Konrad Wothe/Getty Images

Fungi: Basic facts

All types of fungi can be apportioned to one of two groups: yeasts and moulds. Fungi differ from bacteria in many ways, such as they require some source of carbon in order to survive. For example, they can live on decomposing wood and plants and therefore play an important role in the world's ecosystem.

Fungi are also very resilient and can withstand conditions that bacteria cannot. For instance, moulds grow easily on bread, which is usually a dry environment unsuitable for bacterial growth. This type of mould has been beneficial in the medical world due to the power of the penicillin contained within it. It is well known that penicillin formed the basis for the first type of antibiotics ever developed.

Table 1.2 summarises the similarities and differences between the two main forms of fungi.

TABLE 1.2 Yeasts and moulds

Yeasts	Moulds
Found on the outside of plants and fruit	Found on stale bread, cheese and some vegetables
Unicellular, mostly oval in shape and have a cell wall	Multicellular, distinguished by the appearance of long filaments called hyphae
Usually larger in size than bacteria	Usually larger in size than bacteria
Mostly reproduce in an asexual manner	Mostly reproduce in an asexual manner
A common yeast infection is caused by *Candida albicans*, and is known as 'thrush'	A common mould is *Penicillium*, also known as penicillin. These particular moulds create specific chemicals that produce the antibacterial properties within the antibiotic we now know as penicillin

Fungi: Naming structure

The naming structure of fungi has been based on the type of reproduction it relies upon. Since fungi can reproduce both sexually and asexually, there has been a dual naming system in place that has caused some confusion. Fungi are based on the same naming system as bacteria, whereby they have two names; for example, *Candida albicans*.

Fungi: Morphology

This group of microorganisms is extremely diverse in both appearance and morphology. Fungi are comprised of filaments (called hyphae) whereby their cells are elongated and strand-like but connected from end to end (see **Figure 1.5**). Due to the complexity of their cells, a body of fungi is called a mycelium. Once reproductive hyphae are created, they form a large organised structure called a sporocarp, which is more commonly known as a mushroom. This is produced only for the release of spores as it is not the living growing part of the fungus.

Fungi: Classification

Fungal infections are referred to as a form of **mycosis** and are further classified by the location on the body; for example, a commonly known fungus is tinea, which is termed acutaneous mycosis (cutaneous referring to the skin). Although there are hundreds of different types of fungi, only about 100 species actually cause harm to humans.

Example of a fungal infection: Tinea pedis

Tinea pedis, commonly known as tinea, is a fungal infection specifically affecting feet. It prospers in warm and humid environments. The people most susceptible to contracting tinea pedis are young men and athletes.

Tinea pedis is most frequently caused by the following types of fungi:

- *Trichophyton (T.) rubrum*
- *T. interdigitale*, previously called *T. mentagrophytes* var. interdigitale
- *Epidermophyton floccosum.*

Symptoms of tinea pedis

Tinea pedis presents only on the feet and particularly between the toes. This area is usually inflamed and often has patchy areas that are flaking or peeling. The other hallmark symptom of tinea pedis is a sense of itchiness and burning.

Transmission of tinea pedis

Tinea pedis thrives and spreads easily in warm, damp environments such as damp sporting footwear, communal showers and other humid locations such as pool areas. People who do not wear shoes in communal showers and pool areas are prone to spreading and contracting the fungal infection.

Susceptibility of tinea pedis

It stands to reason that people who frequently engage in sporting and aquatic activities are the most likely candidates for acquiring tinea pedis, especially if they repeatedly forgo footwear.

However, if a localised infection such as tinea pedis manages to spread throughout the whole body, it is then considered to be a systemic fungal infection. However, this usually only occurs in people who already have a compromised immune system.

Clients undergoing treatments such as chemotherapy and transplant recipients have weakened immune systems and the fungi can take advantage of this. These types of complications are known as opportunistic infections, which will be discussed at length later in this chapter.

Diagnosis of tinea pedis

A diagnosis of a fungal infection can only truly be determined by collecting a swab for testing. Largely, clinicians will determine a fungal infection based on the presentation of signs and symptoms. In cases of tinea pedis the signs and symptoms, as mentioned above, are often universally distinct and readily identifiable to the experienced clinician.

Treatment of tinea pedis

An anti-fungal cream such as Canestan (clotrimazole) (**Figure 1.6**) will reduce the presence of the fungus, limit reproduction and transmission while also alleviating the irritating symptoms. In addition, it is advised to take preventive measures to avoid re-infection such as:

- wearing shoes or at least thongs in communal settings
- ensuring that footwear is adequately air dried between uses
- ensuring that footwear and socks (preferably cotton to allow the feet to 'breathe') are thoroughly clean prior to use
- scrupulously drying between the toes after showering or swimming.

FIGURE 1.6 A common topical treatment for fungal infections includes the use of a cream such as clotrimazole

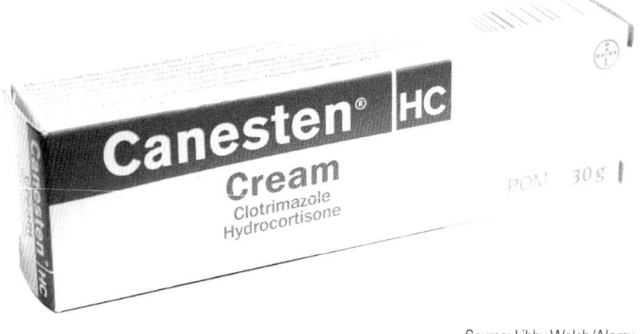

Source: Libby Welch/Alamy

Viruses

A virus is a microorganism that cannot replicate without a host cell. It asserts its power by attaching genetic material into the host cell and takes over its function. In this way, it is able to control the host cell, and as such cause the symptoms commonly seen when someone experiences a viral infection.

Viruses: Basic facts

Viruses are known to be the smallest microorganisms capable of causing infection. They are very different from the other microorganisms previously discussed. Viruses are unique because they only need one type of genetic information for replication; that is ribonucleic acid (**RNA**) or deoxyribonucleic acid (**DNA**).

In addition, viruses are not considered living organisms because they require another cell to invade in order to live and replicate. This cell that supplies the virus with the necessities for survival is therefore called the host cell.

Viruses are unique in many ways and have certain distinguishing features. Viruses are particular about which host cells they choose to invade. Generally speaking, human viruses will only invade humans and animal viruses will only invade animals. However, there are exceptions to this rule, such as the Hendra virus, which will be discussed later in the chapter.

The infective process involves the virus entering a host cell and quickly replicating itself, thus rendering the host cell defenceless. Once the host cell is completely dominated and overpopulated by the virus, the virus breaks through the host cell wall and continues to target other host cells and the whole cycle begins again.

Viruses: Naming structure

The naming structure for a virus is similar to the other microorganisms already discussed. The species name is usually drawn from the actual virus itself. It starts at the level of order and continues as follows:

- order
- family
- sub-family
- genus
- species.

Viruses: Morphology

While viruses also vary in morphology, they are relatively simple in structure compared with their counterparts. While most are spherical in shape there are a few exceptions, such as:

- the rhabdovirus is a bullet-like shape
- the poxvirus (the largest virus of all) is a brick-like shape
- the bacteriophage is a tadpole-like shape
- the tobacco mosaic virus is rod shaped.

Viruses: Classification

Viruses are largely classified by characteristics such as:

- morphology
- nucleic acid type
- nature of replication
- types of host organisms
- most importantly, the specific kind of disease they cause.

Some argument exists about the classification of viruses due to the debate of whether or not a virus constitutes a living entity, as viruses can only survive while reliant on a host cell. At present, there are two main systems for the classification of viruses:

- the International Committee on Taxonomy of Viruses (ICTV)
- Baltimore classification system.

However, it is not the aim of this discussion to closely examine these classification systems.

FIGURE 1.7 This figure depicts a basic overview of the anatomy of the respiratory system, which is commonly where viruses thrive and present symptoms

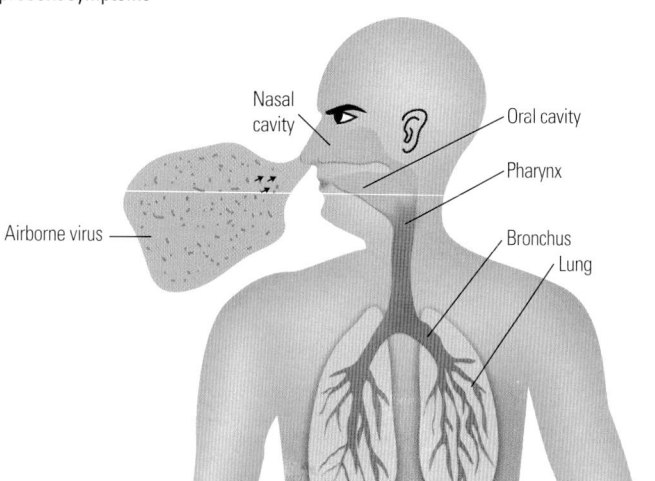

Viruses: Symptoms

While it would be impossible to cover all symptoms of all viruses in this discussion, it is worthwhile to list some of the generalised symptoms. The most common viral symptoms occur in the respiratory tract system (see **Figure 1.7**) and can often present as:

- sore throat
- difficulty breathing

- blocked nose
- increased production of secretions
- fatigue
- fever
- headache.

Viruses: Transmission

There are two types of transmission processes for most infectious agents and viruses also follow this format. Mostly, transmission is from one person to another, which is referred to as horizontal transmission; the second process is from mother to baby and is called vertical transmission.

For most infectious transmission processes, there are three main modes for transportation:

- direct/non-direct contact
- droplet
- airborne.

These modes of transmission will be discussed at length in Chapter 2.

Viruses: Susceptibility

The people most susceptible to contracting a viral infection are no different from those discussed in the MRSA susceptibility section on page 6. As for most infections in a healthy person, the immune system would take charge by producing **antibodies** against the infection and therefore eradicating it. At times, even a healthy person can succumb to an infectious agent such as a virus.

While the immune system produces its own antidote to eradicate many viruses, this process is actually what creates the symptoms associated with a viral infection.

Viruses: Diagnosis

Viral diagnosis can be performed in a number of different ways, including sending a sample to the laboratory for testing. This also includes blood tests that can detect the presence of specific viral antibodies, which are produced in response to the viral infection process.

Viruses: Treatment

It is important to note that the treatment of a viral infection usually only includes addressing the symptoms, such as rest and medications to reduce fever and pain. Unlike bacterial infections, viruses are resistant to antibiotics and therefore once an illness is established as viral, antibiotics are not prescribed. Occasionally, antibiotics are prescribed even when an illness has been established as viral. This is because of the increased likelihood of a secondary bacterial infection because the immune system is already under strain.

Example of a virus: The Hendra virus

The Hendra virus (primarily affecting horses) first identified in Brisbane, Queensland, is one instance where a virus can be transmitted from animals to humans. Primarily this is because there are particular host cells ideal for viral replication common to both the horse and the human.

Symptoms of the Hendra virus

The Hendra virus initially produces flu-like symptoms including fever, cough, fatigue and aches and pains. In many cases, these symptoms progress and can lead to fits, loss of consciousness and eventually death.

Horses can display signs and symptoms that involve the respiratory tract, such as a cough or increased nasal secretions, alongside nervous system impairment. According to the Australian Veterinary Association, there is up to a 70 per cent death rate for horses with these symptoms that also had a confirmed case of Hendra virus.

Transmission of the Hendra virus

The transmission of the Hendra virus is thought to be linked to horses that have become infected by flying fox droppings or secretions. This could be through eating grass that has been contaminated with flying fox bodily fluids.

Susceptibility to the Hendra virus

People working closely with horses, such as trainers and strappers, are highly susceptible to exposure to horses' bodily secretions due to frequent handling and cleaning of stables. Similarly, horse owners, vets and those who work in horse-oriented workplaces are also highly susceptible to the Hendra virus for the same reasons.

Diagnosis of the Hendra virus

Diagnosis is established via blood samples that look at specific antibodies commonly found in those infected with the virus.

Treatment of the Hendra virus

Although there is now a Hendra virus **vaccine** available for horses to prevent the infection, there is no known vaccine for humans. However, some recent clinical trials conducted by the Centers for Disease Control and Prevention have found that a medication called ribavirin has proven helpful in treating the virus, but evidence is not conclusive, especially in humans. Visit http://www.cdc.gov/ > CDC A–Z Index > H > Hendra Virus Disease (HeV) > Resources: Fact Sheet (PDF).

Dormant viruses

Occasionally there are small components of a virus that the immune system does not completely eradicate, even though symptoms have gone and recovery is evident. This is because some small particles of viruses can 'rest' in other cells of the body

that are not actually host cells. No replication occurs and therefore the person is asymptomatic, but the virus is able to lie **dormant** for lengthy periods.

The varicella-zoster virus is a common example of how a virus can remain dormant for decades and then be reactivated, including triggering presentation of viral signs and symptoms.

The varicella virus, commonly known as chickenpox, has historically had a high prevalence of infection in school-aged children. Once the virus is managed and eradicated effectively by the immune system, it has the ability to lie dormant in certain cells of the body.

In times of significant compromise to the immune system, for example, as a person moves into their older years, the virus can be revitalised and start invading the appropriate host cells to cause a related infection, herpes zoster, commonly referred to as shingles. Similar to chickenpox, shingles can produce skin lesions, which can be infectious; it can also attack and inflame the nervous system pathways, causing serious nerve pain.

ACTIVITY

Hendra virus transmission prevention

List three ways that a horse trainer could protect themselves and reduce the likelihood of contracting the Hendra virus.

Parasites

A **parasite** can be described as an organism that survives and proliferates from others while contributing nothing to the host organism for its wellbeing. Parasites can be divided into two distinct groups: **protozoa** and **helminths**.

Protozoa

Protozoa include all of the so-called acellular or unicellular forms of parasites and consist of a single functional cell unit or aggregation of non-differentiated cells, loosely held together and not forming tissues.

An example of a protozoal infection is *Giardia*, which will be discussed later in this chapter.

Protozoa: Basic facts

Most protozoans are found in water or have some involvement with it; for example, mosquitos are perfect vehicles as they aid in the reproduction of protozoa by favouring water sources and then transferring some protozoa to humans via biting and accessing the blood supply; however, some common wild and domesticated animals as well as some other insects also act as satisfactory vehicles. All three of these **habitats** can be possible **reservoirs** for transmission to humans and therefore pose a threat to general wellbeing and even a person's life.

Although many protozoa thrive in polluted water, such as in developing countries, there have been cases in Australia where clean and treated water have become contaminated, causing significant harm to people. This is largely attributed to system anomalies in the treatment and detection of protozoans in our water systems. It is interesting to note that protozoans are far more resilient in the water treatment process than bacteria and they are difficult to detect and measure. Therefore, it is easy to see why they pose a threat to humans.

Survival and reproduction of protozoa are reliant on the consumption and immersion of tiny molecules such as food or other microscopic organisms within their surrounds. Some protozoa have clearly distinguished gullets, similar to a fish, while others gain their nutrients via a process called phagocytosis. This means that the protozoa can swallow their nutrients by completely surrounding them and incorporating them into the protozoal cell.

Protozoa: Naming structure

The naming structure for protozoa is the same as for bacteria; see page 2.

Protozoa: Morphology

Protozoa are single-celled microorganisms and therefore fall into the eukaryotic classification. Unlike most other microorganisms, they do not contain a cell wall; rather they are only protected by a robust cell membrane.

Although only a single-celled organism, the protozoa contains small organelles that can also be found in other organisms, such as bacteria. For example, some protozoa have hair-like projections on the outside of the cell membrane, called flagella, that are used for moving.

Protozoa: Classification

Lee and Bishop (2010) have identified that protozoa are classified in accordance with how they move and can be separated into four main groups:

- Sarcodina (**amoebae**) – this type of protozoa has the ability to enlarge its cell membrane to allow the **cytoplasm** (the large component within the cell wall) to contour itself into a foot-shaped appendage to propel itself.
- Mastigophora (flagellates) – these protozoa can mobilise themselves easily due to their tail-like appendages, flagella, which are especially useful in water-based environments.
- **Ciliates** – this particular protozoa has hair-like appendages that move in synchronous fashion for quick and easy movement.
- **Sporozoa** – unlike the other types of protozoa, this type does not have any appendages to create movement. It is entirely motionless. (Lee and Bishop, 2010, p. 117).

Protozoa: Symptoms

Symptoms of protozoan infections will differ depending on the specific type of protozoa concerned and also which body system is most likely to be affected by it. Here is a list of some generalised symptoms potentially indicative of a protozoan infection:

- fever
- flu-like symptoms
- nausea
- vomiting
- abdominal pain
- rectal bleeding
- abdominal bloating
- increased heart rate.

Protozoa: Transmission

Protozoan transmission is facilitated by any one of four main modes:

- direct – from person to person from close contact (e.g. unprotected sex)
- faecal–oral route – where infected faeces are accidentally ingested
- vector-borne – when infected insects transmit, especially to humans via biting
- predator–prey transmission – when a predator eats infected prey.

Protozoa: Susceptibility

The people most susceptible to contracting a protozoal infection are the same as those already discussed in the MRSA susceptibility section on page 6.

Protozoa: Diagnosis

Most diagnoses are based on the detection of symptoms, but there is also standardised faeces testing available. The emergence of newer technology has recently allowed for more extensive faecal analysis and therefore more accurate diagnostics.

Protozoa: Treatment

Treatment is prescribed based on the particular type of protozoa identified during the diagnosis stage. There are effective medications to treat and resolve protozoal infections, but they can be difficult to treat if diagnosis and identification is not established.

Example of a protozoal infection: *Giardia*

Giardia intestinalis (*Giardia lamblia*) is a water-borne microorganism that favours the digestive tract for survival and reproduction. Untreated water is the most common reservoir for these protozoa prior to entering the host.

Although it is quite common in developing countries where clean water can be difficult to access, it is also present in Australia and even in highly populated and urbanised areas. In 1998, it was discovered that Sydney's water supply had become contaminated with both *Giardia* and *Cryptosporidium*.

Symptoms of *Giardia* infection

As mentioned, this protozoa ideally flourishes in the digestive tract and so most signs and symptoms of infection will be related to this body system. Common symptoms include stomach pain, diarrhoea, weight loss and fatigue; however, these are somewhat vague and hence diagnosis can be problematic.

Transmission of *Giardia*

As *Giardia* is water-borne parasite it is common for transmission to be oral, that is, through drinking contaminated water. This is not limited to accidental contamination of drinking water, but can also include fresh water streams and stagnant dams. In addition, it can also be transmitted via food, especially if fruits and vegetables are washed with local contaminated water in locations such as in developing countries.

Susceptibility to *Giardia*

Those people who travel to countries where clean drinking water is unavailable are at risk of contracting *Giardia*. People who spend time in the bush and are therefore more likely to swim in dams or drink from streams also place themselves at risk. Also, those who already have a pre-existing digestive problem may be at heightened risk of contracting *Giardia*, especially if they engage in the high-risk activities previously mentioned.

Diagnosis of *Giardia*

Although diagnosis is difficult and treatment is often only partially successful, there are specific tests that can be performed by examining the person's faeces. If a clinician is in doubt about a conclusive diagnosis, and there are protracted periods of symptoms, the recommended medication for *Giardia* is often prescribed.

Treatment of *Giardia*

The most common medication for treating *Giardia* is Flagyl (metronidazole), and if it reduces or eliminates the *Giardia* symptoms, then it is usually deemed a successful treatment.

Helminths

The other type of parasite is the group called helminths. Helminth is a general term for a worm. Although there are many different types of worms, they can be distinguished by their classification, largely pertaining to their prefixes. The list on page 20 provides a detailed example about the actions of Helminths, but is only concerned with nematodes as these are the only types of helminths found in humans.

Helminths: Basic facts

They are commonly known as worms and are multicellular eukaryotic microorganisms made up of different cells performing specific functions for survival.

Helminths: Naming structure

The naming structure for helminths is the same as for bacteria; see page 2.

Helminths: Morphology and classification

There are three main sub-groups of helminths, as listed in **Table 1.3** opposite.

TABLE 1.3 Morphology and classification of helminths

Morphology title	Description	Picture
Cestodes (also known as tapeworms)	They are divided into parts including a distinct head and body. The head has little suckers that can easily latch onto a host's intestines, whereby there is a ready supply of nutrients for survival. These are most commonly seen in dogs.	Source: Jubal Harshaw/Shutterstock
Trematodes (also known as flukes)	They are flat and frond shaped. They have a very basic kind of digestive system including a mouth. Similar to the cestodes, they also have suckers that can easily attach to the host's flesh for survival purposes. The most common host is a specific breed of snail and it is not common in Australia.	Source: Carolina Biological/Visuals Unlimited/Corbis

Morphology title	Description	Picture
Nematodes (also known as hookworms, threadworms and roundworms)	These are tubular in shape and, although they do not have clearly segmented sections like the other helminths, they do contain a complete digestive system with mouth, digestive tract and rectum. These are the most common forms of worms found in children.	 Source: Dr. Arthur Siegelman/Visuals Unlimited/Corbis

Helminths: Symptoms

Symptoms of helminth infections will differ depending on the specific type of worm concerned and also which body system is most likely to be affected by it. Generalised symptoms potentially indicative of a helminth infection are:

- nodules under the skin
- conjunctivitis
- retinitis
- blindness
- itching, especially of the skin
- diarrhoea
- cough
- wheeze
- liver dysfunction
- fever
- abdominal pain.

Helminths: Transmission

There are four main vehicles of transmission for helminths where the larvae infect new hosts. These include:

- faecal–oral – as mentioned in protozoal transmission on page 16. Family pets transmit helminths to humans via the faecal–oral route
- transdermal – when infected larvae in soil penetrate the host's skin and move to the gut to create new eggs that are excreted in faeces
- vector-borne – as mentioned in protozoal transmission on page 16
- predator–prey transmission – as mentioned in protozoal transmission on page 16. This includes the ingestion of non-processed or incorrectly processed meat products.

Helminths: Susceptibility

Most people are susceptible to contracting a helminth-based infection. Susceptibility is the same as discussed in the MRSA susceptibility section on page 6.

Helminths: Diagnosis

Diagnosis is determined through the same processes outlined for protozoa on page 16.

Helminths: Treatment

Treatment is prescribed based on the particular type of helminth identified during the diagnosis stage. There are effective medications to treat and resolve helminth infections, but they can be difficult to treat if diagnosis and identification is not established.

Example of a helminth infection: Worms

The most common worms affecting people are roundworms, hookworms and threadworms.

Symptoms of worms

The primary symptom of the presence of worms is anal itching due to localised irritation. This is more commonly experienced at night because that is when the female worms lay their eggs around the anal area.

Transmission of worms

The most significant route of transmission in this instance is oral ingestion as children are prone to putting their hands in their mouths and/or not effectively washing their hands after scratching. Naturally, most children will want to scratch the area to provide relief, but in doing so they also transfer eggs onto their hands, under their fingernails and onto bedding.

Susceptibility to worms

At some stage, most school-aged children contract worms and this group is the most susceptible to infection. Once the eggs enter the digestive system they are able to successfully feed off the host's gut and reproduce effectively. After defecation, the whole cycle starts again with the worm laying eggs and the child scratching the anal area. Hence, it is difficult to eradicate worms in children due to the ongoing nature of the cycle.

Diagnosis of worms

At times, it may be possible to see worms either around the anus or in the faeces and therefore confirmation and diagnosis of worms is obvious. However, if this evidence is not apparent, it may be necessary to conduct a test whereby a special type of tape is pressed against the anus to collect any eggs that may be present. This is sent to pathology for further testing and verification of diagnosis. In some cases, a faecal specimen may be required to ensure accurate identification of the suspected worm.

Treatment of worms

The treatment of worms is relatively easy as appropriate oral medication can be purchased over the counter at most pharmacies. There are some exceptions to this and some medications do require a script from a clinician.

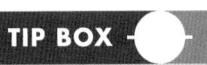

TIP BOX

Treating worm infestations
It is very important that the whole family be treated at the same time as the infected child, alongside any bedding and clothing that may have been affected.

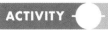

ACTIVITY

Childhood worms

List three ways to prevent the occurrence and recurrence of childhood worms.

Resident and transient flora

All people have a certain amount of microorganisms on and in their body that are generally of little clinical consequence and normally cause no harm. This is referred to as normal flora and can include many different types of bacteria.

There are many different types of normal flora and each type favours particular sites on and in the body (see **Table 1.4**). This is referred to as resident flora; for example, the normal flora in the digestive system would not normally be found on the skin. While the digestive system flora remains inside its own domain, it usually causes no harm to any other body system.

Similarly, there are flora that can be present for short periods, usually on the skin and especially the hands of healthcare workers, which can be quite easily reduced or removed. This is called transient flora and is commonly managed by effective and frequent handwashing techniques. The clinical focus on transient flora concerns mainly the hands, as they are among the greatest carriers of microorganisms in a healthcare setting.

Broadly speaking, it is only when a person's normal flora transfers to a foreign site in the body that there is potential for infection.

TABLE 1.4 Summary of the normal flora and the usual locations on the body

Location	Normal flora	
Mouth	• Staphylococci • Strep. viridans • Enterococci • Strep. pneumoniae • Neisseriae • Corynebacterium • Haemophilus	• Enterobacteriaceae • Actinomyces • Lactobacilli • Bifidobacteria • Fusobacteria • Anaerobic Gram negative cocci
Gastro-intestinal tract	• Helicobacter pylori • Streptococci • Lactobacilli • Candida albicans and other yeasts • Bacteroides	• Bifidobacteria • Eubacterium • Coliforms (e.g. E. coli) • Streptococci • Lactobacilli • Clostridium
Skin	• Staphylococci • Corynebacterium	• Propionibacteria • Anaerobic Gram negative cocci
Vagina	• Staphylococci • Strep. viridans • Enterococci • Neisseriae • Corynebacterium	• Lactobacilli • Bifidobacteria • Bacteroides • Anaerobic Gram negative cocci

There are certain circumstances that can promote the transmission or reduction of normal flora. For instance, factors such as hospitalisation, invasive procedures, surgery, old age, poor nutrition and repeated exposure to common antibiotics can have detrimental impacts on normal flora. In turn, this can lead to infections that are either already resistant to certain antibiotics, or opportunistic infections, which will be discussed in the next section.

Aspects of infectious agents and pathogens

This section will give a brief overview of particular aspects of infectious agents, including actual and potential sources of infection. Other clinically significant aspects of infection include the presence of opportunistic organisms alongside other pathogens. At this stage, these concepts are introduced; they are expanded in Chapter 2.

Endogenous and exogenous causes of infection

Infectious diseases may be classified as **endogenous** or **exogenous**, depending on the source of the causative pathogen.

Endogenous diseases are caused by shift and overgrowth of normal flora. For example, a surgical wound may become infected due to introduction of *Staphylococcus epidermidis*, a microorganism that is classed as normal flora residing on the skin of the client. Due to an interruption of the skin integrity, this usually harmless bacteria is able to infiltrate the body through the surgical wound. The bacteria has then entered the body via a susceptible site, giving it the opportunity to multiply and cause disease. An endogenous infection may also be passed from mother to infant during pregnancy or at the time of birth. Pathogens such as rubella may cross the placenta and cause **congenital** defects.

Exogenous diseases are acquired by exposure to pathogens from the external environment. An example of an exogenous disease could be developing impetigo following a grazed knee sustained from fall in the schoolyard.

Opportunistic organisms

Opportunistic organisms cause harm easily under the right conditions. For example, if a person's immune system is in deficit, then the opportunistic organism will take advantage of this situation and proliferate within the person, causing harm.

However, the organism must find a susceptible host in order to cause disease. There are many factors that may cause a person to become more susceptible to disease than others.

Pre-existing disease

Clients with certain diseases are at a much higher risk of contracting infection caused by an opportunistic organism. Disease processes such as cancer and leukaemia alter the body's capacity to respond to infection. Chronic diseases such as multiple sclerosis (MS), rheumatoid arthritis and diabetes mellitus lead to a general debilitation and therefore increased susceptibility to opportunistic organisms.

As the names suggest, **human immunodeficiency virus (HIV)** and acquired immune deficiency syndrome (AIDS) directly affect the client's ability to maintain an effective immune system. Clients living with HIV and/or AIDS are therefore at significant risk of experiencing an opportunistic infection.

Age – infants and older adults

It is widely accepted that the very young and the elderly are at heightened risk for infection. Babies and young children have immature immune systems. Infants who are breastfed receive antibodies through breast milk from their mother; though clearly beneficial, breast milk alone is inadequate to protect the child from all infections.

Older adults also experience a decrease in their immune response. This may be caused by certain medications (steroids such as prednisone suppress the immune system) or the ageing process itself. As a person ages, bodily changes and deterioration lower their ability to fight infection as well as create occasion for imbalances in natural flora. Skin structure thins and is damaged, easily presenting opportunity for infection. The urinary system may begin to lose its ability to function as competently as previously. Pooling of urine in the bladder leads to increased opportunity for normal flora to multiply, creating imbalance and producing urinary tract infections.

Medications

Some medications and associated therapies are employed specifically to depress the immune system.

Organ transplant recipients require lifelong treatment with **immunosuppressant** medications to ensure their bodies do not reject the transplanted organs. However, this leaves them at heightened risk of acquiring infection through an opportunistic organism.

Used in the battle against cancer and certain chronic diseases such as rheumatoid arthritis, **cytotoxic** and **chemotherapeutic** medications produce a secondary effect whereby the bone marrow, which is responsible for white cell production, is depressed.

Radiation therapy is utilised in the destruction of cancer cells; unfortunately, it also destroys normal cells and produces bone marrow depression, negatively affecting a client's immune system. Clients receiving both cytotoxic or chemotherapeutic medications and radiation therapy are, at times, at such elevated risk of infection they require isolation to protect them from opportunistic infections.

Nutritional status

Clients experiencing poor nutritional intake are more susceptible to infection and may experience a slower rate of healing In particular, protein, carbohydrate and certain fats are essential for an adequate immune system and the healing process. Postoperative clients and clients who have sustained severe extensive burns have increased need for an adequate nutritional intake to promote healing and protect against opportunistic infections.

> **TIP BOX**
>
> **Illness and immunity**
> If unwell, it is always best to avoid contact with people who experience lower levels of immunity.

Pathogens

A **pathogen** is a microorganism or biological agent that is the cause of infectious disease. People exposed to a pathogen may respond in vastly different ways, depending on the state of their immune system and the virulence of the pathogen. For example, a fit healthy young adult with a robust immune system may experience exposure to a pathogen yet avoid developing symptoms of the disease. Equally, an older person or a very young child may experience exposure to the same pathogen and develop disease that may cause their death. Still others may encounter colonisation by the pathogen yet remain free from disease symptoms. Lastly, as we are all mostly familiar with, some people will contract an illness after an asymptomatic period of incubation/colonisation following exposure to a pathogen.

CASE STUDY

Infection transmission processes

Jai Carlisle is in the orthopaedic ward of the hospital following a motorbike accident three days prior. Jai sustained one deep laceration to his right lower leg, which was cleaned and stitched in the operating theatre the morning following his accident. The enrolled nurse, Kathleen, observes Jai's leg bandages are wet with ooze from his wound.

'It started to really throb through the night and I feel awful and really hot', Jai reports.

His temperature is 39.1°C.

Kathleen and the registered nurse, Marie, remove Jai's dressings to find the wound very red and swollen with a large amount of exudate (discharge) in the dressings. Marie takes a swab of the ooze to send to pathology and Kathleen cleans and redresses the wound.

During the doctor's rounds, the surgical registrar states, 'It seems like you have an infection in your wound. We will start you on some antibiotics through an intravenous line. Most likely the infection has either come from a microorganism entering the laceration at the time of your accident or from the resident flora on your skin.'

The results of the wound swab show *Staphylococcus aureus* to be the microorganism causing Jai's infection.

Questions

1 List three signs or symptoms that suggest Jai's wound is infected.

2 Why is a swab being sent to pathology and what is the significance of this?

3 The doctor has suggested that the infection has infiltrated the wound either at the time of injury or from Jai's own skin flora. Define these two different types of infectious processes.

4 What impact would the antibiotics have on the infection?

5 List three signs or symptoms that would indicate the infection is resolving.

- Microorganisms are divided into two groups according to their structure and function – eukaryotic and prokaryotic.
- Bacteria are classified according to their shape, Gram staining qualities and acid-fast staining qualities, and then further identified by genus, species and strain.
- Bacterial infections can be treated by antibiotics, but viruses cannot.
- All fungi are eukaryotic and can be divided into yeasts and moulds.
- Viruses are one of the smallest microorganisms and can lie dormant in their host for years. Although viruses are non-responsive to antibiotics, a person can form immunity to specific viral disease through use of a vaccine.
- Parasites, including protozoa and helminths, are organisms that require a host to live in or on.
  - Protozoa are single-celled eukaryotic organisms
  - Helminths are worms and are categorised into three main subgroups.
- Resident flora are microorganisms that live on or in the body but do not generally cause disease. Transient flora include microorganisms that live on the body for a short time and do not cause disease in normal circumstances.
- Both resident and transient microorganisms have the ability to become pathogenic when there is a disturbance to the body, such as a break in skin integrity from a lesion or wound.
- Opportunistic organisms refer to microorganisms that do not usually cause disease but can become pathogenic under certain circumstances.
- Patients exposed to pathogens may respond in vastly different ways.

REVIEW QUESTIONS

1 Describe the differences between eukaryotic and prokaryotic cells.
2 Describe three structural differences between viruses and bacteria.
3 What is a pathogen?
4 Which microorganism can be treated with antibiotics?
5 List five factors that can increase a client's susceptibility to infection.
6 Explain how an opportunistic microorganism can cause disease.
7 What is the difference between endogenous and exogenous infectious diseases?
8 What defines a parasite?

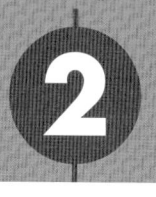

2 DISEASE TRANSMISSION

Introduction

Healthcare facilities, whether they are acute inpatient, slow stream rehabilitation or residential settings, experience ongoing challenges dealing with **healthcare associated infections (HAIs)**. In order to gain control of this ongoing problem, healthcare workers need to understand how infections are introduced to their facility, how to identify the source of infection and who is 'at risk' or presents as a susceptible host for receiving the pathogens and developing an illness. With this knowledge comes the ability to introduce measures that will interrupt the transmission of disease and allow the risk to be effectively managed and so provide optimal protection for the most vulnerable patients.

Paths of disease transmission

For infection to flourish, it is essential that there are three main components working in a collaborative manner. These are a **source of the infection** (previously known as a reservoir), an effective **mode of transmission** and a **susceptible host**.

Source

The infectious process begins with a source, meaning that there is some type of reservoir that enables the microorganisms to grow and thrive. This could be a person, especially one who may be unwell and carrying a pathogen in one or more of their body systems. For example, someone with pneumonia will be carrying a pathogenic microorganism in their respiratory system whereby the person has provided an ideal environment for sustainable replication. Similarly, the source could be within an animal or even medical equipment, food and water. Any of these can potentially become an ideal reservoir for any manner of microorganisms to proliferate.

Mode of transmission

There are three main modes of transmission; these are **contact**, (**direct** or **indirect**), **airborne** or **droplet** methods. In healthcare settings, infection may be transmitted from one person to another by any of these modes.

Contact

Direct contact transmission occurs when direct physical contact transfers microorganisms to a susceptible host via an individual who is either colonised or infected with the microorganism. An example of this is a healthcare worker becoming infected with HIV through direct contact with a client's blood .

Indirect contact transmission occurs when microorganisms are transferred to a susceptible host via an object that has become contaminated. An example of this is the transference of **norovirus** via taps on a hand wash basin used by a person contaminated with the virus.

Penetrating injury transmission of infection takes place when a contaminated object gains entry to a susceptible host via direct infiltration. An example of this is a needle stick injury through to experiencing an impaling injury.

Airborne

Airborne transmission describes organisms that have a true airborne phase in their route of dissemination. This usually results in a distance of more than several feet between the source and the victim. Airborne infections are easily transmitted via dust or droplets in the air and can be disseminated via the following means:

- Coughing, speaking and sneezing will produce droplets (that potentially could contain pathogens) and have the ability to linger in the air and therefore are easily transmitted from person to person.
- Some of these smaller droplets may leave behind nuclei that contain pathogenic particles which have the capacity to remain static in the air for extended periods, thus increasing the likelihood of transmission.
- The presence of dust in the air, on the floor and on items of equipment and other inanimate objects can all trap pathogenic microorganisms and create a gateway for transmission

Pathogens that are transmitted in this way include **varicella** (chicken pox) and **tuberculosis** (TB).

Droplet

In droplet transmission, the infectious agents are expelled from respiratory secretions by coughing, sneezing or talking; this is another form of contact transmission. Droplets are large particles that rapidly settle on horizontal surfaces or are deposited on a susceptible person's conjunctivae, nasal membranes or mouth. They cannot be transmitted beyond a radius of several feet from the source. Pathogens that are transmitted in this way include the common cold virus, influenza viruses and respiratory syncytial virus (RSV). See **Figure 2.1** on page 28 to gain a better understanding of these routes of transmission.

Susceptibility of a host

Chapter 1 introduced the concept of the susceptible host and opportunistic organisms (see page 22). It is far easier for

FIGURE 2.1 Contact, droplet and airborne modes of transmission

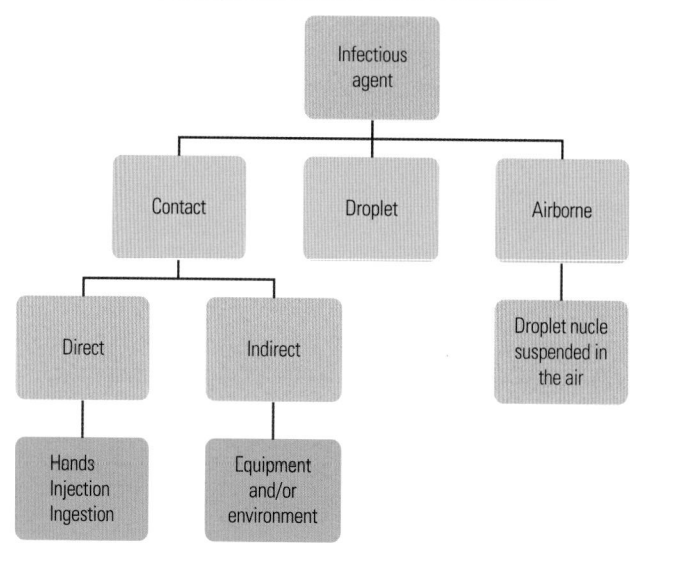

to eradicate it), as well as clients undergoing cancer treatments such as **chemotherapy** and **radiotherapy** that are well known to depress the immune system.

In addition, other medical conditions and contributing factors can affect the immune system, such as **diabetes**, the use of medically-indicated steroids and cigarette smoking. Last, the elderly and the newborns also carry a heightened susceptibility due to generalised immune system compromise.

In a healthy person, the immune system would take charge by producing antibodies against a virus and therefore eradicating it. Although all people are at risk of infection, some groups have increased susceptibility due to varying factors. In particular, the young, the elderly and those with a compromised immune system can quickly become debilitated by an infection.

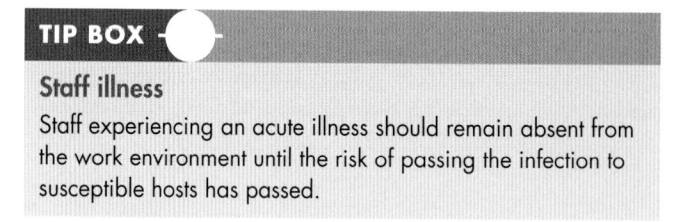

TIP BOX

Staff illness
Staff experiencing an acute illness should remain absent from the work environment until the risk of passing the infection to susceptible hosts has passed.

Young children

Very young children experience heightened susceptibility to acquiring infection, chiefly due to their underdeveloped immune systems. Babies receive some bolstering of immunity while being

pathogenesis to occur when there is a waiting, susceptible host. In particular, the clients we care for are often the most susceptible to infection. Susceptibility springs from some kind of deficit in the body's overall functioning. This may include those who already have a known immune system deficit, such as those who have received organ transplants (recipients receive medications to suppress their immune system so that the body doesn't identify the new organ as a foreign body and attempt breastfed due to the antibodies contained in mothers' breast milk. Childhood immunisation commences on the day of birth with hepatitis B immunisation. A further hepatitis immunisation is received at two months of age. Because they have an underdeveloped immune system, newborn babies should follow the immunisation regimen detailed in the example below.

EXAMPLE

The immunisation regimen for a newborn baby

- Day of birth: hepatitis B
- Two months of age: hepatitis B, diphtheria, tetanus, acellular pertussis (whooping cough), *Haemophilus influenza* type b, inactivated *poliomyelitis* (polio), pneumococcal conjugate and rotavirus
- Four months of age: hepatitis B, diphtheria, tetanus, acellular pertussis (whooping cough), *Haemophilus influenza* type b, inactivated *poliomyelitis* (polio), pneumococcal conjugate and rotavirus

Effectively, newborns do not have any form of immunity to most diseases prior to two months of age, when the immunisation regimen commences. Therefore, newborns rely on the community's herd immunity to protect them when vulnerable. This means that due to widespread immunisation programs across Australia, almost every person has acquired immunity to these diseases via vaccinations. When reservoirs of infection are destroyed, such as

via mass immunisation programs, only the most susceptible people are at risk of contracting a disease but, with herd immunity in place, the risks are extremely low, even for the most susceptible.

An example of herd immunity in Australia is a newborn under two months of age who is generally well protected even in the presence of multiple visitors because the visitors are usually fully immunised. See **Figure 2.2**.

FIGURE 2.2 **Newborn babies rely on herd immunity**

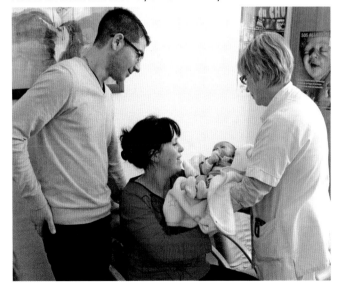

Source: BSIP SA/Alamy

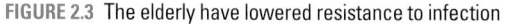

TIP BOX

Herd immunity and the newborn

With the current resurgence of pertussis (whooping cough) in Australia, it is common for parents to request that visitors repeat or check the status of their immunisations prior to visiting their newborn to ensure that herd immunity is in place for the protection of their child.

The elderly

Older people are generally at elevated risk for acquiring an infection and they often experience a more severe course of the related illness (see **Figure 2.3**). Factors contributing to increased susceptibility include:

- 'ageing' or weakened immune system
- chronic age-related disease or multiple chronic conditions
- polypharmacy
- lowered nutritional status

TIP BOX

Outbreaks in aged care

Residential aged care facilities present increased challenges if an infectious disease is introduced to their community. All staff must be aware of the steps that must be taken *immediately* if an outbreak is suspected.

FIGURE 2.3 The elderly have lowered resistance to infection

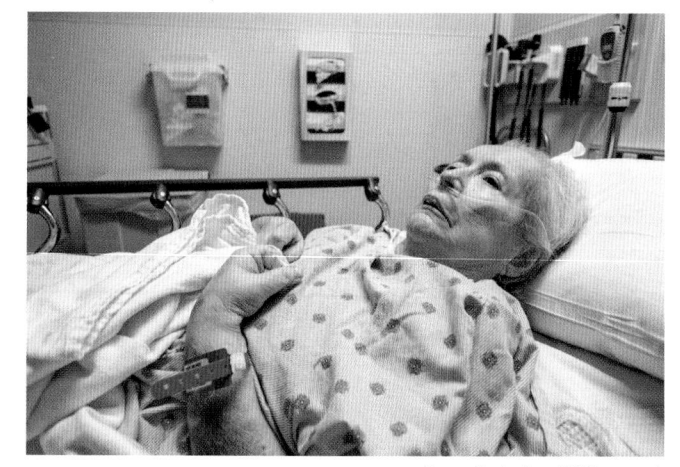

Source: Fotoluminate LLC/Shutterstock

- weakened initial defences – possible breaks in skin integrity
- decreased mobility.

The immunocompromised

As previously mentioned, someone receiving special medications, known as anti-retrovirals, to ensure that the immune system does not reject a newly transplanted organ is deemed as **immunocompromised**. In other words, their immune system has been artificially suppressed for the purposes of ensuring that the new organ is accepted by the body. These clients are therefore considered to be susceptible to infection due to their compromised immune systems. Clients need to be fastidious with ensuring that the other segments of the infection chain are well managed; that is, that exposure to the source or reservoir of infection is eliminated or minimised and that transmission processes are dealt with in the same manner.

Within the category of the immunocompromised client also comes those who experience auto-immune diseases such as diabetes, HIV, ulcerative colitis and multiple sclerosis. Also affected are those receiving chemotherapy and radiotherapy, whereby the treatments incidentally depress the immune system by decreasing the white blood cell production and therefore rendering the body less able to fight infection (see **Figure 2.4**).

Lastly, those clients receiving steroidal-based medications (e.g. prednisone) for inflammatory conditions such as asthma or arthritis also experience a similarly depressed immune system from the active ingredients of the treatment.

TIP BOX

Asthma and candidiasis
People living with asthma and receiving steroid treatment are prone to oral thrush (candidiasis) as the natural balance of flora is disturbed, providing the opportunity for candida to thrive beyond it's usual level of colonisation.

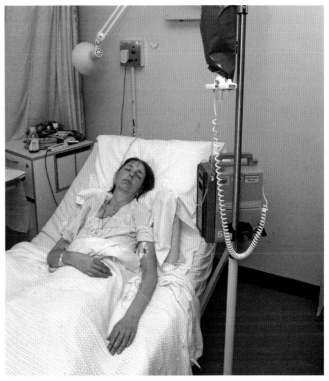

FIGURE 2.4 People receiving chemotherapy or radiation therapy are at very high risk of contracting infections due to their immunocompromised status

Source: CaptureItOne/Alamy

CASE STUDY

Infection risks

Mrs Hutchinson lives in the hostel section of the local nursing home. She is excited that her family are arriving today to celebrate her birthday in the communal dining area with all of her friends from the hostel.

After the party, Mrs Hutchinson experiences violent vomiting and diarrhoea. She is assisted with personal hygiene care and encouraged to drink water as tolerated.

Scenario 1

The night duty enrolled nurse (EN) hands over that Mrs Hutchinson needs to be reviewed by her GP this morning as she seems to have contracted food poisoning. Mrs Hutchinson is feeling very weak but has agreed to go to breakfast to have a cup of tea.

During handover a care worker enters the office, stating, 'Mrs Blackall is vomiting now. She went to Mrs Hutchinsons' party, she's probably got food poisoning as well'. Mrs Blackall is placed on the list for the GP to review when he arrives. 'See if she would like to come to the dining room for a cup of tea. Don't allow her to isolate in her room.'

Scenario 2

The night duty EN hands over that Mrs Hutchinson needs to be reviewed by her GP this morning. She reports that Mrs Hutchinson has experienced violent vomiting and diarrhoea over night and is very weak this morning. The EN directs that Mrs Hutchinson remains in her room at this stage. She directs care staff to use additional precautions including gowns, gloves and masks until Mrs Hutchinson is proved *not* to be an infection risk to the other hostel residents.

During handover a care worker enters the office, stating, 'Mrs Blackall is vomiting now. She was one of the ladies who went to Mrs Hutchinsons' party'.

The EN decides Mrs Blackall will need to stay in her room and as a precaution directs the staff to treat the situation as a possible outbreak of 'gastro'.

Signage is placed and PPE is provided outside both Mrs Hutchinson and Mrs Blackalls' rooms. The ladies are asked to stay in their rooms and advised that staff will be wearing PPE when attending to them. Dedicated bins, marked 'INFECTIOUS WASTE', are placed in the bedrooms.

Questions

1 Identify strategies that differ between the scenarios.

Scenario 1

a Identify any deficits in the EN's decisions.

b What possible outcomes do you forsee because of these deficits?

Scenario 2

c Identify the strengths in the EN's decisions.

d What possible outcomes do you forsee because of these strengths?

Chain of infection

In order for infection to be transmitted there are certain conditions that must be met. This chain of infection is illustrated in **Figure 2.5**. This chain must experience a disturbance to effectively terminate the transmission of the infections.

FIGURE 2.5 The chain of infection

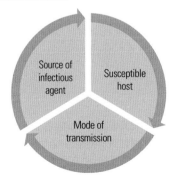

Source: Adapted from 'Australian Guidelines for the Prevention and Control of Infection in Healthcare'. Published by National Health and Medical Research Council (NHMRC), Commonwealth of Australia, © 2010

ACTIVITY

Breaking the chain of infection

In order to decrease episodes of infection, it is necessary to interrupt the chain of infection. Reflect on each of the stages of the chain of infection as listed below. Suggest two interventions you may employ to interrupt each link of the chain of infection.

1 Source of infectious agent

2 Mode of transmission

3 Susceptible host

Risks of disease acquisition

All people entering a healthcare facility can be at risk of acquiring an infection, whether they are staff, patients or visitors. The risk of acquiring an infection can be measured by general indicators and are dependent on the context of the persons' interaction within the environment. For example, a patient requiring complex major surgery will be at a very high risk of acquiring an infection compared with people who may be visiting him in hospital and the staff caring for him. Surgical patients generally are at elevated risk of infection due to disruption in their skin integrity (surgical wound). Similarly, other patients with an interruption to their **integumentary system,** such as traumatic wounds, burns or rashes, will be vulnerable to acquiring infectious diseases usually via the contact route.

Within the general population there are groups of people who are historically at elevated risk of acquiring infections. As previously mentioned, these groups include the very young, the very old, those living with chronic illnesses and those, who for varying reasons, have a compromised immune system. This will be discussed later in the chapter.

Decreasing the risk of disease acquisition

There are general guidelines that help to decrease a person's risk of acquiring a HAI. These are outlined in **Table 2.1**.

TABLE 2.1 Decreasing the risk of healthcare acquired infections

General guidelines for reducing the risk of HAI	
Manage diabetes	Ensuring blood glucose levels are well controlled reduces the risk of acquiring or the severity of an infection.
Quit smoking	Smoking slows the healing process and increases risk for stasis pneumonia and other lung infections.

General guidelines for reducing the risk of HAI	
Practise effective handwashing	Effective handwashing will significantly lower the risk of infection. This applies to all people within the healthcare environment – staff, visitors and patients.
Aim for a healthy weight	People who are either overweight or underweight can be prone to infection.
Ensure your doctor is aware of your recent or current illnesses	Having a head cold may lead to a chest infection if you experience a decrease in mobility secondary to a surgical procedure.
Avoid overuse of antibiotics	Frequent use of antibiotic therapy when possibly unnecessary will lead to an increase of **resistant bacteria.**
Other factors which contribute to the acquisition of disease but are less manageable by the patient	
Admission to a high-risk area	These include intensive care units and high dependency units.
Use of invasive equipment	Indwelling or **suprapubic catheters,** **intravenous** or **central lines, endotracheal** or **tracheostomy tubes,** as well as feeding tubes (both naso-gastric (NG) and **percutaneous endoscopic gastrostomy** (PEG)).
Surgery	The nature of the surgery and length of the operation can influence acquisition of infection.
Length of hospital stay	A person admitted for multiple or complex illnesses may be at increased risk of infection.

Sources and carriers of infectious agents

The source of an infection is where the infection has come from. As previously stated, this could be a person, animal, object or substance. Interestingly, the terms 'source' and 'reservoir' are often used interchangeably, although there are subtle differences. The actual person, animal, object or substance is considered the reservoir for infection while the source could be water or food that enables a mode of transmission. However, there are also many instances where the reservoir and source are the same entity and this is when confusion can play a role. Nonetheless, the three main domains will be briefly discussed.

Human reservoir

The most significant reservoir in the healthcare setting is the human body. Those clients who are unwell are likely to be producing pathogens and transmitting them throughout the environment. Unfortunately, many clients will be able to transmit pathogens while still in the asymptomatic or incubation period, meaning that precautions to minimise the spread of infection will not have been implemented. It is not only asymptomatic clients who enable the ready transmission of pathogens; those clients who may be **carriers** of chronic infections, including **latent viruses**, but remain asymptomatic on presentation also allow transmission.

In addition, the human body can also be its own worst enemy at times. For example, many common infections such as a **urinary tract infections** (UTI) (often referred to as a bladder infection) arises from the body's own reservoir. The bacteria *Escherichia coli* (*E. coli*) is part of the body's normal count of 'good' bacteria, collectively known as flora. *E. coli* is part of the gut's normal flora and functions for the good of the body in the colon. However, when normal flora such *E. coli* move outside their designated environment, it can easily become a potential pathogen for the body when entering other areas. If *E. coli* accidentally enters the urinary tract system (which is relatively easy if a woman wipes from back to front after passing urine) it can cause an infection as it is not part of this system's normal flora.

Animal reservoir

Both domestic and feral animals have the potential of being reservoirs of infection. It is possible that some animals that act as a reservoir can infect humans, even when the animal is asymptomatic. For example, the avian flu virus that can cause disease in birds has been proven to infect humans who handle diseased birds.

Interestingly, many of these types of diseases require a **vector** as a mode of transmission between animal and human. Tapeworm is a vector that easily moves from cattle into humans via the consumption of their infected meat. Similarly, **toxoplasmosis** may be transmitted from the domestic cat to humans via inhalation or even accidental ingestion of cat faeces, especially when cleaning cat litter trays.

Non-living reservoirs

Bodies of water and soil can provide excellent breeding grounds for many types of microorganisms. For instance, *Clostridium tetani* is commonly found in soil and is a very robust microorganism as it can sustain its spores for lengthy periods in the ground by living in excreted faeces. Often, humans are infected with this bacteria when they are accidentally injured (resulting in a break in the skin) by an affected item concealed in the ground.

Similarly, Gram negative pseudomonas are able to flourish on plants and flowers and therefore are easily transmitted to a healthcare setting when well-meaning visitors bring flowers in to brighten a client's day. Unfortunately, this particular bacteria is resistant to many antibiotics and poses a significant threat to those who are most susceptible including those clients in the intensive care unit (ICU), burns victims and those who have had major surgical interventions and/or devices.

It is ill-fated but a real issue that drinking water can easily become contaminated by faeces. Although this is less of a concern in Australia due to stringent water treatment initiatives, it is commonplace in developing countries. Water contamination by faeces is the greatest cause for many infectious diseases in humans, including typhoid, cholera, polio and hepatitis A.

The box on this page contains examples of infection drawn from the differing modes of transmission and reservoirs.

EXAMPLE

Clinical examples of infection from different modes of transmission and varying reservoirs

- A person with a respiratory infection such as *tuberculosis* broadcasts infectious *droplets* through coughing and sneezing.
- Surgical wounds can easily become infected if normal flora from the skin (e.g. *Staphlococcus epidermis*) enters the compromised site via *direct contact*.
- There have been several cases of humans contracting *Hendra virus* via *droplet* transmission from infected horses' respiratory secretions or blood. To date there have been no reported cases of human-to-human transmission.
- Common objects such as hand rails or taps on hand basins that have viral or bacterial infective contamination (usually by previous *indirect contact* with a person experiencing disease symptoms from illnesses such as *norovirus*).
- Bloodborne infections such as human immunodeficiency virus (*HIV*) can be contracted via a needle stick injury (*direct contact*).
- *Giardia* can be contracted from drinking contaminated water acting as a *non-living reservoir* for infection in developing countries such as Nepal.
- *Tetanus* can be contracted by a penetrating injury (*direct contact*) such as stepping on a rusty nail.

Carriers of infection

People who are infected with a disease may be known as carriers. Carriers can be divided into distinct groups:

- The acutely ill
  - While experiencing symptoms of an acute infection such as human swine flu (H1N1), the patient is carrying and shedding infectious particles (see **Figure 2.6**).
- People in the incubation phase of disease
  - This describes the time span between acquiring an infection and displaying symptoms of the disease. Infection can be unknowingly broadcast during this phase. See 'Incubation period of measles' example below.
- Some individuals who have been exposed to an infectious agent may have no symptoms; however, they are still capable of carrying and spreading the infectious agent.
  - For example, 80 per cent of people who have hepatitis C are asymptomatic following contraction of the virus.

FIGURE 2.6 Spread of respiratory infection via droplet mode of transmission

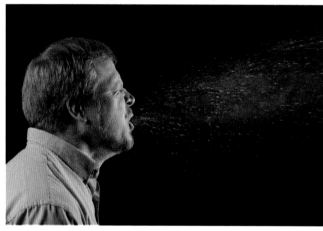

Source: Centers for Disease Control - digital version copyright Science Faction/Science Faction/Corbis

EXAMPLE

Incubation period of measles

Measles (rubeola) has an incubation phase of approximately 10 days; however, this can vary from seven to 18 days from exposure to the onset of fever. The measles rash usually appears 14 days following exposure. Cases can be infectious from five days before the rash appears and up to four to five days following the rash's appearance. The virus can persist in the environment for up to two hours. Transmission has been reported by people whose only apparent source of infection was a room, presumably contaminated with the measles virus when it had been occupied by a patient with measles up to two hours earlier.

SUMMARY

- To effectively reduce episodes of infection, it is important to understand the paths of disease transmission.
- Equally, it is essential to acknowledge and understand the varying risks and factors that contribute to disease acquisition.
- In order for an infection to proliferate, there must be a source or reservoir to enable the process.
- Some people are more susceptible than others to infection and those most at risk include young children and the elderly.
- The risk of disease acquisition in a healthcare facility is dependent to a large extent on the context of interaction of the person within the healthcare environment.
- The risk of disease acquisition can be decreased by following some general guidelines.
- In order to decrease episodes of infection, it is necessary to interrupt the chain of infection.
- Reservoirs for infectious diseases can be both living and non-living entities.

REVIEW QUESTIONS

1 Name three steps in the chain of infection.
2 List five lifestyle factors that can be detrimental to your health.
3 Identify the main modes of infection transmission.
4 What is a susceptible host and which groups of people are at increased vulnerability for acquiring an infection?
5 Name three health promotional activities you are aware of in your community.

6 Reflect on three issues regarding access and equity difficulties you may have experienced in your life.
7 Provide one example of disease spread by each mode of transmission.
8 Explain the concept of 'herd immunity'.

3 IDENTIFYING AND RESPONDING TO INFECTION RISKS

LEARNING OBJECTIVES

At the end of this chapter, you will be able to:

- identify infection control risks in line with organisational infection control frameworks
- understand risk management principles
- adhere to specific infection control protocols
- understand waste management issues in relation to infection control
- understand and use communication of infection control policies and procedures.

Introduction

This chapter aims to provide an understanding of the identification and response processes relating to infection risks in a healthcare setting. The role of individual workers, the concerns of management and how these two forces can collectively address issues of infection control are considered. Specific risk control measures that are commonplace in many healthcare settings are examined in detail. Finally, waste management issues alongside policies and procedures are addressed in the workplace context.

Identifying infection control risks

All members of the healthcare team are responsible for the identification of infection risks. Most healthcare services advocate a systematic approach that includes an infection control framework to ensure overarching consistency and accuracy of responses.

Surveillance programs

A significant part of the framework includes the implementation of an infection control surveillance program to reduce healthcare acquired infections (HAIs). All team members can contribute to the **surveillance** of infections even if simply by collecting data.

According to the **National Health and Medical Research Council (NHMRC)** *Australian Guidelines for the Prevention and Control of Infection in Healthcare* (2010, p. 221) surveillance programs enable:

- the collection of data to establish baseline information on the prevalence and type of infections
- the identification of where and when in the infection control chain infections are enabled to proliferate
- the implementation of appropriate infection control measures to address the exact source and transmission of identified infections.

Most surveillance programs use a combination of strategies to capture vital data, including those concerned with process and those pertaining to outcomes of infection control issues.

Process surveillance

Process surveillance is related to auditing clinical practice against set benchmarks such as policies and procedures that draw from contemporary evidenced-based resources.

A common example of process surveillance is the monitoring and auditing of effective handwashing to improve hand hygiene practices. The **World Health Organization (WHO)** has produced hand hygiene assessment tools for use in clinical areas that emphasise evaluation and outcomes. Visit http://www.who.int/ > Programmes > Clean Care is Safer Care > Save Lives: Clean Your Hands and look for tools.

Similarly, Hand Hygiene Australia also has numerous tools for hand hygiene audits and compliance. These include but are not limited to the utilisation of technology such as The Hand Hygiene Compliance Application (App) for use on mobile phones. See http://www.hha.org.au/ > Hand Hygiene Compliance Application – HHCApp > HHCApp_WHO for further details.

Outcome surveillance

Outcome surveillance focuses on critical incidents that have occurred and examines the contributing factors in its development. This approach is aimed at detecting previous adverse events concerning infection and preventing recurrence, especially where mortality is concerned.

At times, different **healthcare workers (HCWs)** will be required to contribute to outcome surveillance programs and any subsequent changes in practice that may be required for future prevention of infections.

Working within frameworks

The ability to identify infection control risks in a clinical setting and a working knowledge of the correct response to the problem is directly linked to the role of the healthcare worker. That is, the designation of the worker will dictate varying levels of response in the implementation of control procedures.

While there may be some problems that can only be addressed by management, such as changes in policies and procedures in order to rectify or reduce risks, there are many issues that are within the scope of practice of the HCW. This includes positions such as **assistants in nursing (AINs)**, **personal care workers (PCWs)** (also known as personal care assistants), **allied health workers (AHWs)** and **enrolled** and **registered nurses** (ENs and RNs). Collectively, the entire team can contribute to the process of identifying actual and potential infection risks while implementing processes in accordance with the facility's infection control framework.

It is an expectation that all staff – including AINs, HCWs, PCWs, AHWs, ENs and RNs – will contribute to and participate in these types of process audits to identify areas for improvement in practice.

Understanding risk management principles

Communication and consultation are important aspects of risk management. An information exchange between management, healthcare workers and clients will assist in increasing awareness of infection prevention and control, and prompt identification and management of risks.

Alongside the surveillance programs is a systematic framework to identify, assess and respond to infection risks in a clinical setting. In particular, the Australian/New Zealand standard on risk management, AS/NZS ISO 31000:2009, provides a user-friendly framework that also promotes continuous quality improvement. This is in accordance with the hierarchy of control of infection and is advocated by infection control experts. See Figure 3.1 to gain an understanding of the process.

The hierarchy of control

The hierarchy of control is based on risk reduction measures that are ordered in priority for implementation purposes. See Table 3.1 on page 42 to better understand the application of these measures, which may be used concurrently to achieve the best possible outcome.

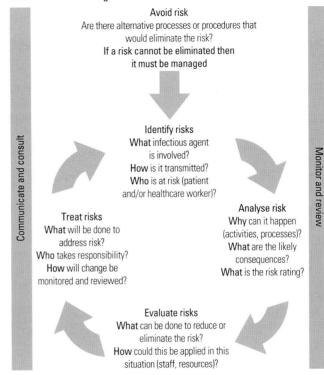

FIGURE 3.1 Risk-management flowchart

Avoid risk
Are there alternative processes or procedures that would eliminate the risk?
If a risk cannot be eliminated then it must be managed

Identify risks
What infectious agent is involved?
How is it transmitted?
Who is at risk (patient and/or healthcare worker)?

Analyse risk
Why can it happen (activities, processes)?
What are the likely consequences?
What is the risk rating?

Evaluate risks
What can be done to reduce or eliminate the risk?
How could this be applied in this situation (staff, resources)?

Treat risks
What will be done to address risk?
Who takes responsibility?
How will change be monitored and reviewed?

Communicate and consult

Monitor and review

Source: National Health and Medical Research Council (NHMRC) (2010). *Australian Guidelines for the Prevention and Control of Infection in Healthcare.* http://www.nhmrc.gov.au/book/australian-guidelines-prevention-and-control-infection-healthcare-2010/a2-2-risk-management-pro

TABLE 3.1 Hierarchy of control in regards to risk reduction

Control measure	Applying a control measure
Elimination	Wherever it is possible, it is always better to eliminate the risk presented.
Substitution	If elimination is not realistic, consider the possibility of substituting an item or practice for another that may significantly reduce the risk.
Isolation	In order to protect the general public, consider isolating the hazard by restricting access to pertinent staff members only.
Engineering controls	If possible, consider the re-design of certain pieces of equipment that are potential hazards.
Administrative controls	Ensure that policies, procedures, practices and guidelines are aimed at minimising risk. Educate staff about how to avoid or best manage the risk.
Personal protective equipment	Provide equipment designed to protect the individual from the hazard and thus minimise risk.

ACTIVITY

Applying hierarchy of control and the risk analysis matrix

Using the hierarchy of control (in **Table 3.1**) and the risk analysis matrix (in **Table 3.2**), apply these principles to the following scenario:

You are working a morning shift in a residential aged care facility. Before you start for the day, you walk into Mr Bonski's room to find the following concerns:

- urine on floor (catheter bag accidentally left open)
- a used needle left in a kidney dish on the client's bedside table
- clinical waste bin overflowing.

In compiling your response you may find it useful to place information in a box with headings, such as the example provided below.

Identified risk	Level of risk	Risk reduction measure
Urine on floor		
Used needle		
Clinical waste overflowing		

In order to identify the risks in the first instance, many facilities have also used the NHMRC Risk Analysis Matrix tool to establish the probability and severity of risk concerned. See **Table 3.2** for details.

TABLE 3.2 Risk analysis matrix

Consequences

Likelihood	Negligible	Minor	Moderate	Major	Extreme
Rare	Low	Low	Low	Medium	High
Unlikely	Low	Medium	Medium	High	Very high
Possible	Low	Medium	High	Very high	Very high
Likely	Medium	High	Very high	Very high	Extreme
Almost certain	Medium	Very high	Very high	Extreme	Extreme

Low risk Manage by routine procedures.

Medium risk Manage by specific monitoring or audit procedures.

High risk
Very high risk
Extreme risk
This is serious and must be addressed immediately.
The magnitude of the consequences of an event, should it occur, and the likelihood of that event occurring, are assessed in the context of the effectiveness of existing strategies and controls.

Source: National Health and Medical Research Council (NHMRC) (2010). 'Part A: Basics of Infection Prevention and Control' (p. 24). *Australian Guidelines for the Prevention and Control of Infection in Healthcare.* http://www.nhmrc.gov.au/book/australian-guidelines-prevention-and-control-infection-healthcare-2010/part-basics-infection-pr

Adhering to specific infection control protocols

In order to better understand how the risk management flowchart and the associated analysis matrix relate to practice, it is useful to apply it to particular clinical incidents. The following discussion will explore protocols for use when exposed to blood and body fluids and also following spills, in accordance with the policies and procedures of the organisation.

Protocols following exposure to blood and bodily fluids

Due to the nature of healthcare delivery, there will always be inherent risk to staff in relation to exposure to blood and body fluids. Therefore, it is vital that all staff are aware of both risk reduction strategies and the specific protocols to follow in the event of exposure.

TIP BOX

Needle stick injuries
Ninety-eight per cent of staff who suffer a needle stick injury from a known hepatitis C carrier will not become infected.

While it is usually a requirement of employment that clinical staff are vaccinated against some of the significant pathogens found in blood and body fluids, it is important to also know that standard precautions and prescribed protocols must also be implemented. Clinical staff can be easily exposed to bloodborne pathogens such as:

- hepatitis B and C (HBV and HCV)
- human immunodeficiency virus (HIV, which can progress to acquired immunodeficiency syndrome [AIDS])
- measles, mumps and rubella
- diphtheria, pertussis and tetanus.

Therefore, it stands to reason that standard precautions are always maintained.

The next part of the discussion outlines typical examples of how a healthcare worker can be exposed to blood and body fluids.

Needle stick injury from giving an injection

Either prior to giving an injection or after administration, especially in the disposal stage, it is possible for a HCW to prick themselves with a needle. Obviously, if the injury occurs after administration when the needle is 'dirty', then the risks of contracting an infection or disease are heightened. This is known as a *needle stick injury.*

Emptying an indwelling catheter

It is possible for urine to splash in a HCWs *eyes* when emptying an **indwelling catheter (IDC)** bag if correct **personal protective equipment** (PPE) is not used (e.g. goggles). Furthermore, should the HCW have a break in their skin integrity and the wound is not covered, it is possible that urine could splash into it, causing a significant exposure to bodily fluids.

Removal of sterile drapes after surgery

After surgery there will be sterile drapes that have become soaked in blood or bodily fluids during the operation.

During the cleaning-up process after surgery, most clinicians have taken off their masks (which were used to protect the patient, not the HCW) and, especially if in a rush, blood or body fluids can potentially be splashed into the *mouth* of a HCW.

Giving a patient a blood transfusion

During the process of preparing, administering and completing a blood transfusion, it is possible that the HCW could accidentally receive a splash into their *mouth*, even with the correct use of PPE, as most facilities advocate the use of goggles, gowns and gloves but rarely the use of face masks.

Providing first aid

While PPE is effective in reducing exposure to blood and body fluids, there could be circumstances that are not anticipated, such as an arterial bleed that spurts onto a HCW's *skin*, such as the lower leg or arm that may not be covered with PPE at the time. In this instance, exposure to a patient's blood can be a risk even if the skin is intact. However, it is of greater significance if there is a break in the skin, especially if it is not protected by a dressing.

Dealing with a patient who has an acute mental health issue

A patient who is experiencing mental distress for whatever reason may express feelings of anger toward the HCW. It is possible that the patient could bite the HCW, inflicting superficial tissue damage to the *skin*. Although not a huge risk to the HCW, there is still a risk of exposure to **bloodborne viruses** (BBVs).

Attending to a patient's personal hygiene

Patients who are bed-bound, cognitively impaired, resistive or aggressive and also incontinent pose a challenge to the most skilled HCW. In these circumstances it is possible that the HCW could be exposed to faeces, especially if the patient is experiencing diarrhoea. The act of washing a patient, changing sheets and replacing clothing and pads can all lead to accidental splashes into the *eyes* and *mouth*, particularly when a patient is resistant to care.

Prevention and treatment protocols following exposure to blood and bodily fluids

In most healthcare environments, exposure to blood and bodily fluids such as needle stick injuries are common but almost entirely preventable by following the correct organisational policies and procedures. Similarly, adverse effects from such exposures can be significantly minimised by following organisational protocols. The following discussion outlines the prevention strategies and treatment protocols following adverse exposures.

Prevention of exposure

Organisations are obliged to provide specific education surrounding the safe disposal of sharps and avoiding exposure to blood and bodily fluids. This is accompanied by supporting policies and procedures. For example, many organisations will make it a policy that when administering an injection, a sharps bin must be taken to the patient's bedside. This ensures that the sharp is disposed of immediately after use and into the correct receptacle, rather than carried back to the medication room, which would provide the opportunity to slip, trip or fall with the sharp in the hand.

Furthermore, many organisations use retractable needles as an adjunct to the prevention of needle stick injuries.

Almost all organisations advocate via policy the correct usage of PPE when there is potential for exposure to blood and bodily fluids.

Treatment after exposure

The treatment after exposure to blood and bodily fluids is typically the same for any organisation. Authorities on this matter will follow almost identical protocols.

The Centre for Healthcare Related Infection Surveillance and Prevention (CHRISP) has provided the following protocols for the 'immediate care of the exposed person':

Immediately following exposure to blood or body fluids, it is recommended that the exposed person undertakes the following steps as soon as possible:
- wash wounds and skin sites that have been in contact with blood or body fluids with soap and water
  - apply a sterile dressing as necessary, and apply pressure through the dressing if bleeding is still occurring.

- do not squeeze or rub the injury site
- if blood gets on the skin, irrespective of whether there are cuts or abrasions, wash well with soap and water
- irrigate mucous membranes and eyes (remove contact lenses) with water or normal saline
  - if eyes are contaminated, rinse while they are open, gently but thoroughly (for at least 30 seconds) with water or normal saline
  - if blood or body fluids get in the mouth, spit them out and then rinse the mouth with water several times
- if clothing is contaminated, remove clothing and shower if necessary.

When water is not available, use of non-water cleanser or antiseptive should replace the use of soap and water for washing cuts or punctures of the skin or intact skin. The application of strong solutions (for example, bleach or iodine) to wounds or skin sites is not recommended.

For human bites, the clinical evaluation should include the possibility that both the person bitten and the person who inflicted the bite were exposed to BBVs.

Source: Centre for Healthcare Related Infection Surveillance and Prevention (CHRISP) & Tuberculosis Control (2014). *Guideline for the management of occupational exposure to blood and body fluids.* (p. 2). Queensland Health. http://www.health.qld.gov.au/qhpolicy/docs/gdl/qh-gdl-321-8.pdf

If an individual sustains wounds contaminated with other hazards, such as with soil, their tetanus status should be established (refer to the current edition of the *Australian Immunisation Handbook* for more information).

Further management strategies for the treatment and management required after exposure to bodily fluids is illustrated in **Figure 3.2**.

FIGURE 3.2 Guidelines for the management of blood and body fluid exposures

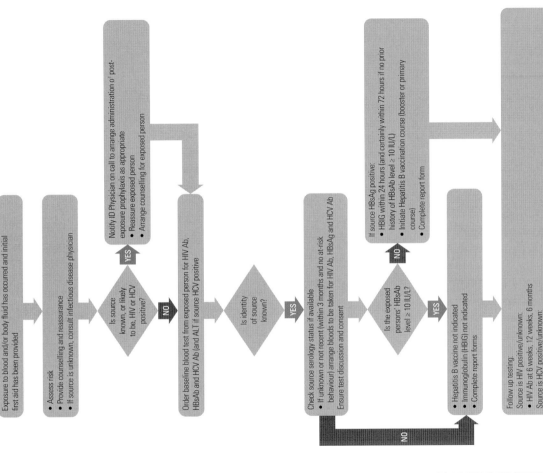

Exposure to blood and/or body fluid has occurred and initial first aid has been provided

↓

- Assess risk
- Provide counselling and reassurance
- If source is unknown, consult infectious disease physician

↓

Is source known, or likely to be, HIV or HCV positive?

YES →
Notify ID Physician on call to arrange administration of post-exposure prophylaxis as appropriate
- Reassure exposed person
- Arrange counselling for exposed person

NO ↓

Order baseline blood test from exposed person for HIV Ab, HBsAb and HCV Ab (and ALT if source HCV positive

↓

Is identity of source known?

YES →

Check source serology status if available
- If unknown or not recent (within 3 months and no at-risk behaviour) arrange bloods to be taken for HIV Ab, HBsAg and HCV Ab
Ensure test discussion and consent

↓

Is the exposed persons' HBsAb level ≥ 10 IU/L?

NO →
If source HBsAg positive:
- HBIG within 24 hours (and certainly within 72 hours if no prior history of HBsAb level ≥ 10 IU/L)
- Initiate Hepatitis B vaccination course (booster or primary course)
- Complete report form

→

YES →
- Hepatitis B vaccine not indicated
- Immunoglobulin (HBIG) not indicated
- Complete report forms

NO (from "Is identity of source known?") →

Follow up testing:
Source is HIV positive/unknown:
- HIV Ab at 6 weeks, 12 weeks, 6 months
Source is HCV positive/unknown:
- HCV Ab and ALT at 12 weeks, 6 months
- If HCW performs EPP, earlier and more frequent follow up may be required — seek advice from Expert Information Network
- HCV RNA indicated if follow up test positive for HCV Ab &/or elevated ALT
If source negative for HCV, HIV:
- No further testing generally required
If exposed person is not immune to HBV at time of exposure, no prior history of HBsAb ≥10 IU/L and source HBsAg positive/unknown:
- LFT at 6 weeks and 12 weeks
- HBsAg at 12 weeks and 6 months [may give a false positive if tested within 2 weeks of giving Hepatitis B vaccine]
- If exposed person immune (HBsAb level ≥10 IU/L) at time of exposure, follow-up for Hepatitis B not indicated

Source: Adapted from Centre for Healthcare Related Infection Surveillance and Prevention & Tuberculosis Control (CHRISP) (2014). *Guideline for the management of occupational exposure to blood and body fluids.* (p. 15).
© The State of Queensland (Queensland Health)

Protocols following spills

The healthcare environment lends itself to unintentional incidents such as spills, including bodily fluids and ordinary substances such as food and drinks. The most commonly spilt substance is water, which could be from any manner of activity, including cleaning equipment such as mops and buckets.

When a spill does occur it is important to assess the risk of the incident and carry out rectifications in line with organisational procedures. This includes establishing whether or not it is a bodily fluid spill or not. Most organisations will have differing procedures for spills that contain bodily fluids and those that do not. The steps for how to effectively manage blood or bodily fluid spills are outlined below.

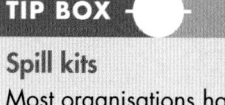

TIP BOX

Spill kits
Most organisations have pre-packed spill kits available. Make sure you know where they are located.

Managing a minor splash/spill of a few drops of bodily fluid

Step 1   Place the A-frame safety sign near the spill. The sign should alert others that a spill has occurred or at least that the floor is wet.

Step 2   Gather PPE including gloves, apron, mask, goggles and rubbish bag. Put on PPE.

Step 3   Place paper towel or something similar that is disposable over the spill.

Step 4   Place paper towels in rubbish bag and place in contaminated waste immediately.

Step 5   Remove PPE and perform hand hygiene. Inform the person in charge and complete the organisational documentation as required; for example, most facilities have an incident form to note the detail of the incident.

Step 6   Remove A-frame sign once it has been established that the area is dry and ready to walk on.

Managing a minor spill of bodily fluid (up to 10 cm in diameter)

Step 1   Follow steps 1–3 as above.

Step 2   These types of more substantial spills can be best dealt with by a more robust paper towel (if available) rather than the standard ones available near hand washing facilities.

Step 3   Place the paper towels into a heavy duty container or waste bag.

Step 4   Wash the area with hot soap and water, again using disposable items.

Step 5   Wipe the area over with sodium hypochlorite (also known as bleach).

Step 6   Place the remaining rubbish items into the container or bag and dispose of into the contaminated waste immediately.

Step 7 Remove PPE and perform hand hygiene. Inform the person in charge and complete the organisational documentation as required; for example, most facilities have an incident form to note the detail of the incident.

Step 8 Remove A-frame sign once it has been established that the area is dry and ready to walk on.

Managing a large spill of bodily fluid (anything over 10 cm in diameter)

Step 1 Follow steps 1 and 2 from the first minor splash/spill section above.

Step 2 Cover the area with a clumping agent such as the absorbent granules included in the spill kit and let sit while it absorbs.

Step 3 Use a disposable scooper to collect the clumping agent containing bodily fluids and place into a heavy duty container and dispose into clinical waste immediately.

Step 4 Mop the area with hot soap and water, followed by cleaning with sodium hypochlorite.

Step 5 Remove PPE and perform hand hygiene. Inform the person in charge and complete the organisational documentation as required; for example, most facilities have an incident form to note the detail of the incident.

Step 6 Remove A-frame sign once it has been established that the area is dry and ready to walk on.

Understanding waste management issues in relation to infection control

According to the NHMRC (2010), there is no widely accepted definition of waste or clinical waste across Australia. However, the Queensland Department of Environment and Heritage Protection defines clinical waste as:

> waste that has the potential to cause disease, including, for example, the following:
> - animal waste
> - discarded sharps
> - human tissue waste
> - laboratory waste.

Queensland Department of Environment and Heritage Protection (2015). *Guideline: Clinical and related waste.* http://www.ehp.qld.gov.au/era/clinical-and-related-waste-em1329.pdf

Other waste is referred to as general waste and includes all other types of rubbish that do not contain bodily fluids. It is standard practice for organisations to apply different protocols for waste management dependent on whether it is considered to be clinical or general waste.

The NHMRC (2010) has advised of the following principles when handling, packaging, labelling, storing, transporting and disposing of waste:
- The generator of the waste is responsible for correct handling, transport and disposal of it.

- All practices must comply with the Australian and New Zealand standard, *AS/NZS 3816:1998 Management of clinical and related waste*. For more information visit http://infostore.saiglobal.com/store/ and enter 'AS/NZS 3816' in the search bar.
- All waste must be managed in accordance with its classification at the point where it is created; that is, waste must be handled and disposed of as soon as possible from the location where it was generated. It would be a significant and unnecessary risk to transport waste to differing locations and handle it again prior to disposal. Abiding by this principle means that correct segregation of waste has been achieved and will enhance safety for storing, transporting and final disposal of waste.
- Correct segregation of waste also means that unnecessary and costly disposal methods can be reserved only for those items at highest risk.

Using personal protective equipment when handling waste

There are several considerations that the HCW must contemplate prior to handling any waste. For instance, a risk assessment should be conducted prior to handling waste to establish whether it is clinical or general waste. This process will enable the HCW to decide the level of risk involved and what type of PPE is necessary.

- Irrespective of the type of waste, always use standard precautions including PPE when handling waste, in accordance with workplace health and safety policies and procedures.
- Clinical waste must be handled with extreme care and only disposed of in the universally recognised yellow wheelie bin, clearly labelled with the words, 'clinical waste' and usually located in a designated 'dirty' area such as a pan room.
- General waste can be disposed of in the closest general waste bin in any area of the facility. General waste bins can always be distinguished from clinical waste receptacles as they are readily available in almost every area, usually white in colour and have no discernible labelling.

ACTIVITY

Using PPE
Consider the following scenario and apply the principles learnt from this chapter to choose the most appropriate course of action.

You have discovered a large spill of blood and contaminated dressings on the floor because a rubbish bag split open during transit. You are aware that you will need to use PPE and a spill kit to clean it up. Outline the sequence of steps you would take and the PPE needed, highlighting the significance of order when donning and removing PPE.

Minimising environmental impacts

The Commonwealth Department of the Environment has the authority to protect the environment including any issues relating to clinical waste management. In order to promote sustainability, the *Waste Avoidance and Resource Recovery Act 2007* was established to protect human health and to also aim towards a waste-free society.

The Environmental Protection Regulations (2004) were implemented to police the transport of clinical waste to avoid accidental release into the environment alongside the prevention of associated health risks. These regulations also provide for the approval and licensing of vehicles and drivers concerned in the transport of clinical waste. Organisational policies and procedures will be embedded by these Acts and Regulations to ensure the overall safety of the handling, transport and disposal of waste.

CASE STUDY

Minimising waste

A new national waste management initiative has been implemented across a variety of industries, including healthcare. Anglicare (a community-based nursing service) in South Australia has joined the campaign to eliminate the production of industry-created waste. The program is called *Zero Waste*.

Anglicare has managed to divert general and clinical waste from landfill sites. In a small timeframe (approximately six weeks) the initiative has increased re-direction and recycling of waste from 20 per cent to 70 per cent.

There are now eight recycling modes including:

✓ cardboard
✓ plain paper
✓ organic material
✓ co-mingled (mixed including glass and plastics)
✓ confidential paper work
✓ clinical waste
✓ sharps (needles)
✓ grease-trap waste.

The one remaining obstacle is the safe and efficient disposal of incontinence pads. Anglicare is committed to overcoming this hurdle and plans to embark upon an Australian-first initiative to prevent pads from choking available landfill.

Questions

1 Consider the issue of incontinence pads and landfill. Suggest a strategy to avoid pads entering landfill.
2 When recycling or otherwise disposing of sensitive identifying documentation, what is the major concern? Suggest strategies to deal with the identified problem.
3 Identify work modifications that may be required to contribute to successful reduction of landfill waste.

Safe storage and disposal of waste

The storage and disposal of waste is followed in accordance with the following legislation:

- *Waste Reduction and Recycling Act 2011*
- Waste Reduction and Recycling Regulation 2011
- Environmental Protection Regulation 2008.

According to NHMRC guidelines, the storage of clinical waste must be a lockable area not accessible to the public. Also, it must have sufficient airflow for proper ventilation, and adequate lighting. In addition, the area must be clearly signposted as a site containing clinical waste.

Communicating infection control policies and procedures

While there has been some discussion of workplace policies and procedures, it is important to remember that these guiding documents need to be discussed, not just read. Team communication about policies and procedures permits time for clarification and understanding connected to the complex issues contained within them.

The following activity will provide you with an opportunity to practise the required skills for communication surrounding policies and procedures.

ACTIVITY

Policies and procedures

You have been asked to introduce the concept of the infection control policies and procedures relevant to your setting to a group of new employees.

In your discussion, include a real-life example drawn from the content in this chapter. For example, discuss how to manage a bodily fluid spill in accordance with your organisation's policies and procedures.

SUMMARY

- Infection control and risk assessment responses are in direct accordance with organisational frameworks and the healthcare worker's designated role. This includes understanding the risk management principles of surveillance, the identification of deficits and the implementation of corrective measures.
- The hierarchy of risk control measures provides a systematic approach for the application of significant changes in infection control policies and procedures.
- The risk analysis matrix can assist in the identification of the likelihood of risk and the level of consequence. Effective risk management is crucial in the minimisation of infection control breaches.
- Safe waste management includes following particular protocols to ensure the safety of all employees and to avoid detrimental consequences to the environment. This includes management of spills and bodily fluid exposure.
- Organisational policies and procedures need to be discussed in a team setting and applied within the clinical environment.

REVIEW QUESTIONS

1 Describe one benefit of an infection control surveillance program.
2 List the top two measures used in the hierarchy of risk control.
3 Name two functions of the risk analysis matrix.
4 Name one significant difference in procedural practice between the management of a body fluid spill and a water spill.
5 Outline the steps involved in the management of a needle stick injury.
6 Describe one simple infection control risk management strategy that you could implement within your role.
7 Discuss two goals surrounding the safe handling, packing, labelling, storage, transport and disposal of clinical waste.

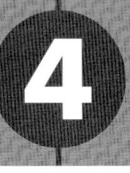

4 FOLLOWING INFECTION CONTROL GUIDELINES

LEARNING OBJECTIVES

At the end of this chapter, you will be able to:

- follow infection control guidelines in a clinical setting
- implement effective hand hygiene practices
- implement personal hygiene practices
- use personal protective equipment (PPE) when indicated
- clean environmental surfaces
- safely handle and dispose of sharps
- ensure sterility of instruments.

Introduction

This chapter outlines the significance of implementing effective infection control guidelines in a healthcare setting. These guidelines include the understanding of standard and transmission-based precautions and when they are clinically indicated. In addition, the implications of correct hand hygiene as well as sound personal hygiene practices are highlighted. Cleaning practices, both routine and also in special circumstances, are linked in with standard and transmission-based precautions. Finally, the guidelines look at the safe handling and disposal of sharps and the sterility of items prior to use.

Infection control precautions

Infection control guidelines in a clinical setting are universal to all health-related workplaces. In particular, there are two basic strategies that form the foundation for successful infection control. These include the application of **standard precautions** and **transmission-based precautions**. When implemented stringently, these two factors have the ability to eliminate sources of infection transmission.

Standard precautions

Standard precautions include all practices, such as those outlined in **Figure 4.1**, that aim to limit or prevent the transmission of infection regardless of whether there is knowledge that it exists or not. When standard precautions were first implemented, clinicians often said it was an approach whereby patients were considered to be infectious, regardless of their actual status. Therefore, this is seen as a protective mechanism to ensure that microorganisms are not transmitted from person to person or any equipment in the clinical environment.

FIGURE 4.1 Standard precautions sign

Standard Precautions

Always follow these standard precautions

Perform hand hygiene before and after every patient contact

Use personal protective equipment when risk of body fluid exposure

Use and dispose of sharps safely

Perform routine environmental cleaning

Clean and reprocess shared patient equipment

Follow respiratory hygiene and cough etiquette

Use aseptic technique

Handle and dispose of waste and used linen safely

AUSTRALIAN COMMISSION
ON **SAFETY** AND **QUALITY** IN **HEALTH CARE**

Source: Australian Commission on Safety and Quality in Health Care (n.d.). 'Approach 3 Standard Precautions Photo'. *National infection control guidelines*. http://www.safetyandquality.gov.au/our-work/healthcare-associated-infection/national-infection-control-guidelines/approach-3-standard-precautions-photo-pdf-693kb/

Table 4.1 provides practical examples of how standard precautions are implemented in a clinical setting.

Transmission-based precautions

Transmission-based precautions are the secondary strategy of infection control in the clinical setting. In particular, these precautions are used when a patient has a known infection and precautions can therefore be structured accordingly to decrease the risk of transmission to others. Transmission-based precautions are also used when there is a particular outbreak, especially in large-scale healthcare settings such as **residential aged care facilities** (RACF) and acute settings such as hospitals.

TABLE 4.1 Standard precautions in practice

Example of standard precaution practice	Rationale or aim of practice
Hand hygiene	This is the single most effective method of reducing transmission of infection in a clinical setting.
Use of personal protective equipment (PPE)	The use of gloves, gowns and protective eye wear aims to limit exposure to bodily fluids, thus limiting transmission of infectious agents.
Correct handling and disposal of sharps	This is to decrease the risk of transmitting infections, especially those that are bloodborne, as sharps nearly always contain bodily fluids.
Correct cleaning/decontamination of reusable instruments and equipment	Non-invasive and reusable pieces of equipment must be thoroughly cleaned between patient use to limit contamination and transmission of microorganisms among patients and healthcare workers.
Housekeeping management	Prompt management of spills and routine cleaning are important for limiting the spread of infections. Correct disposal of general rubbish and contaminated waste also contributes to the reduction in transmission rates. Appropriate management of linen, including contaminated articles, will reduce transmission of potentially infectious agents.
Correct cough etiquette	Covering the mouth while coughing and hygienic disposal of respiratory excretions will significantly reduce the transmission of infections.
Non-touch technique	Careful use of clean hands and equipment will limit the introduction of microorganisms to at-risk sites, especially in regard to patients.

FIGURE 4.2 Isolation of infection

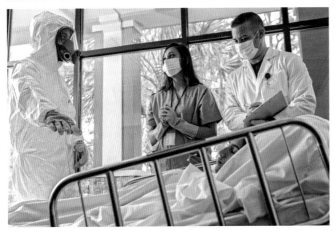

Source: Terry J Alcorn/Getty Images

Table 4.2 illustrates how transmission based precautions are implemented in a clinical setting.

TABLE 4.2 Transmission-based precautions in practice

Example of transmission-based precautions	Rationale/aim/practice
Isolation of infection	Use of single rooms for patients with known infections, to contain transmission. (See **Figure 4.2**) Where single rooms are not available, grouping patients with the same infection together is recommended.
Patient movement	Patient movement within the healthcare setting should be limited to only urgent activities such as lifesaving medical imaging.
Contact precautions (transmitted through touch)	Use of gowns, gloves and goggles would be one way to limit the spread of infection from patient to healthcare worker. Also, using dedicated pieces of equipment for one particular patient will limit the transmission process.
Droplet precautions (transmitted via large droplets, including sources such as talking, coughing and sneezing)	Use of a standard surgical mask will protect healthcare workers and visitors from large droplet contamination from the patient. Similarly, if the patient needs to move out of their room for some reason, then the patient will be instructed to wear the surgical mask to protect others.
Airborne precautions (transmitted via small elements)	Use of a high functioning mask called a P2 respirator will protect healthcare workers and visitors from small elements and gases that could cause infection. (Note: competency in fitting the mask must be undertaken by all users.) If the patient needs to move out of their room, then the patient will be instructed to wear the P2 respirator to protect others. Ideally, a negative pressure room should be provided for patients who require airborne precautions. This will ensure that the contaminated air is not re-circulated to adjacent rooms.

The signs in **Figure 4.3** are the nationally accepted depictions regarding the three different types of precautions taken in healthcare facilities.

FIGURE 4.3 Precaution signs: a) contact precautions

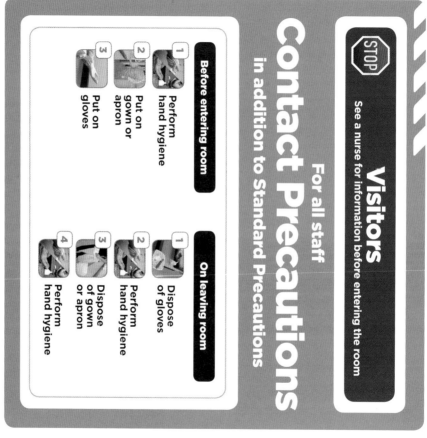

STOP

Visitors

See a nurse for information before entering the room

Contact Precautions

in addition to Standard Precautions

For all staff

Before entering room

1 Perform hand hygiene

2 Put on gown or apron

3 Put on gloves

On leaving room

1 Dispose of gloves

2 Perform hand hygiene

3 Dispose of gown or apron

4 Perform hand hygiene

Standard Precautions

And **always** follow these **standard precautions**

- Perform hand hygiene before and after every patient contact
- Use PPE when risk of body fluid exposure
- Use and dispose of sharps safely
- Perform routine environmental cleaning
- Clean and reprocess shared patient equipment
- Follow respiratory hygiene and cough etiquette
- Use aseptic technique
- Handle and dispose of waste and used linen safely

AUSTRALIAN COMMISSION
ON **SAFETY** AND **QUALITY** IN **HEALTH CARE**

FIGURE 4.3 Precaution signs (continued): b) Droplet precautions

Visitors

See a nurse for information before entering the room

For all staff

Droplet Precautions

in addition to Standard Precautions

Before entering room

1. **Perform hand hygiene**

2. **Put on a surgical mask**

On leaving room

1. **Dispose of mask**

2. **Perform hand hygiene**

Standard Precautions

And **always** follow these **standard precautions**

- Perform hand hygiene before and after every patient contact
- Use PPE when risk of body fluid exposure

- Use and dispose of sharps safely
- Perform routine environmental cleaning
- Clean and reprocess shared patient equipment

- Follow respiratory hygiene and cough etiquette
- Use aseptic technique
- Handle and dispose of waste and used linen safely

AUSTRALIAN COMMISSION
ON SAFETY AND QUALITY IN HEALTH CARE

FIGURE 4.3 Precaution signs (continued): c) Airborne precautions

STOP

Visitors

See a nurse for information before entering the room

For all staff

Airborne Precautions

in addition to Standard Precautions

Before entering room

1. Perform hand hygiene

2. Put on N95 or P2 mask

3. Perform a fit check of the mask

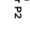

On leaving room

1. Dispose of mask

2. Perform hand hygiene

Keep door closed at all times

Standard Precautions

And **always** follow these **standard precautions**

- Perform hand hygiene before and after every patient contact
- Use PPE when risk of body fluid exposure
- Use and dispose of sharps safely
- Perform routine environmental cleaning
- Clean and reprocess shared patient equipment
- Follow respiratory hygiene and cough etiquette
- Use aseptic technique
- Handle and dispose of waste and used linen safely

AUSTRALIAN COMMISSION
ON SAFETY AND QUALITY IN HEALTH CARE

Using precautions

Read the following scenarios and choose the answer that you think is the most clinically appropriate course of action.

1 You are working in a busy emergency department (ED) and are caring for Mrs Swoski who is suspected of having tuberculosis (TB). After an episode of coughing, she has just placed used tissues on the food table. Choose which of the following precautions should be used:

   a Standard precautions need to be used as well as the provision of a contaminated waste bin.

   b Airborne precautions need to be used as well as thorough decontamination of the food table and the provision of a contaminated waste bin.

   c Transmission-based precautions need to be used as well as sterilisation of the food table.

2 You are working in an aged care residential setting, caring for Mr Kerzig, who is faecally incontinent and requires assistance with personal care.
   Choose from the following which precautions and use of PPE would be most suitable when providing his personal care.

   a Blood and bloodborne precautions with the use of sterile gloves and mask.

   b Droplet precautions with the use of ordinary gloves and full sleeved sterile gown.

   c Standard precautions with the use of ordinary gloves and plastic apron.

Implementing effective hand hygiene practices

Hand hygiene practices form the pillar of infection prevention in most healthcare settings. For some time now, the infection control mantra has been: *handwashing is the single most effective infection control measure taken by healthcare workers in the prevention of transmission of potential pathogens.*

However, it cannot be stressed enough that the technique for handwashing must be strictly followed. Healthcare workers, patients and the community itself need to understand the essential steps to take to conduct an effective handwash process.

There are two specific types of handwashing procedures commonly used in general healthcare settings. The first technique is referred to as a **social or routine handwash** and is used in everyday circumstances to limit the transmission of microorganisms. For example, after a person uses the toilet they wash their hands and this is simply part of routine life.

The other type of handwashing technique is called a **clinical handwash** (see **Figure 4.4** on page 62) and this is used prior to performing invasive procedures such as a dressing. However, it is important to note that it is not the same as the **surgical handwash**, often showcased on TV programs.

The next part of the discussion will provide examples of when handwashing may be applied in a clinical setting and specific information on the different types of handwashing techniques that are used.

FIGURE 4.4 Clinical handwash

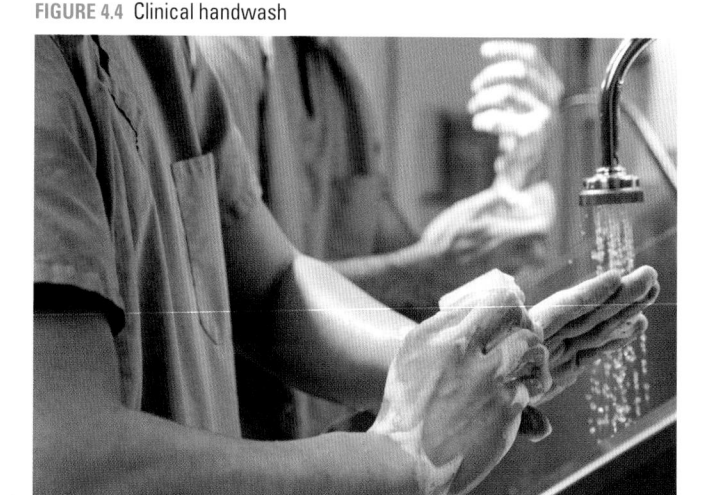

Source: Andersen Ross/Getty Images

A social handwash should always be conducted in the following circumstances:

- Before and after *any* patient contact.
- Before and after commencing duty.
- Before and after meal breaks while on duty.
- When hands are obviously soiled.
- After eating or handling food and drinks, or visiting the toilet.
- After touching/wiping face, nose or mouth.
- After touching inanimate objects such as phones, computers, patient equipment or furniture.
- After handling waste of any kind.
- In the event of contamination by bodily fluids.
- After removal of gloves.

Social handwashing duration and technique

According to WHO (2009), a social handwash should take approximately 40 to 60 seconds in duration. The actual technique of a social handwash should be as follows:

1 When turning on the tap, adjust flow and temperature to comfort but ensure that the water is not hot as this is drying on the skin and can compromise the healthcare worker's skin integrity.
2 Wet hands first and then apply pump soap, ensuring that all areas of the hand are covered in soap.
3 Rub palm to palm, then palm over back of other hand with fingers interlaced.
4 Rub backs of fingers against the opposite palm of hand.
5 Rub up and down both the left and right thumbs.
6 Circular rubbing of each palm with opposing finger tips.
7 Rinse hands thoroughly with fingers pointing in an upwards direction.
8 Use clean paper towel to pat dry hands.
9 Turn tap off with paper towel or elbow if able.

Alcohol-based hand rubs

If hands have not become visibly soiled and the task being performed involves minimal patient contact, such as passing a plate or medicine cup, it is acceptable to cleanse hands with an alcohol-based hand rub (ABHR). However, it must be highlighted that these hand rubs have limited scope and should not be used as a replacement of a hand wash. The technique for use is similar to a social handwash in regards to the rubbing motions but there is no need to dry hands because of the evaporative properties of the alcohol in the product.

Clinical handwash duration and technique

According to WHO (2009), a clinical handwash should last for a minimum of one minute. While the technique for a clinical handwash is the same as above, it is imperative that jewellery is removed. A plain wedding band without any stones is acceptable, but the healthcare worker must ensure that the area under and around the band is thoroughly washed and dried. A clinical handwash is indicated prior to any invasive or potentially invasive procedures, such as before performing a dressing or inserting an indwelling catheter and prior to opening sterile packages.

Surgical handwash duration and technique

WHO (2009) recommends between two and five minutes for a surgical handwash but does not advocate lengthy scrubs of 10 minutes or more. Again, the basic technique remains the same but in a surgical handwash it is necessary to also clean under the finger nails. WHO (2009) does not recommend the use of brushes but does advocate using nail sticks to ensure all foreign particles are removed. In addition, it is strictly prohibited to wear any form of jewellery; this includes a plain wedding band. A surgical handwash in indicated prior to surgery and when assisting in

the operating theatre (OT) in any capacity. It is also indicated when performing high-risk clinical procedures such as accessing central line devices.

Many institutions around the world have recognised the significance of handwashing. See **Figure 4.5** on page 64 for examples of how some organisations across the world are promoting handwashing and highlighting the gravity of the problem.

TIP BOX

Hand hygiene and moisturiser
Hand hygiene does not stop at handwashing alone. It also incorporates the care of the skin on the hands and the importance of good skin integrity. This includes the use of moisturisers on hands throughout the working day and also while off duty.

Personal hygiene practices

Personal hygiene practices are extremely important in the healthcare setting. This includes showering, washing hair and wearing clean uniforms.

While it might seem like commonsense to most of us, it is still important to remind everyone that the personal hygiene of a healthcare worker is no less important than that of the patient. It is essential that workers shower daily and wash hair frequently (e.g. two or three times per week).

FIGURE 4.5 Posters from the Centers for Disease Control and Prevention's *Hand Hygiene Saves Lives* campaign

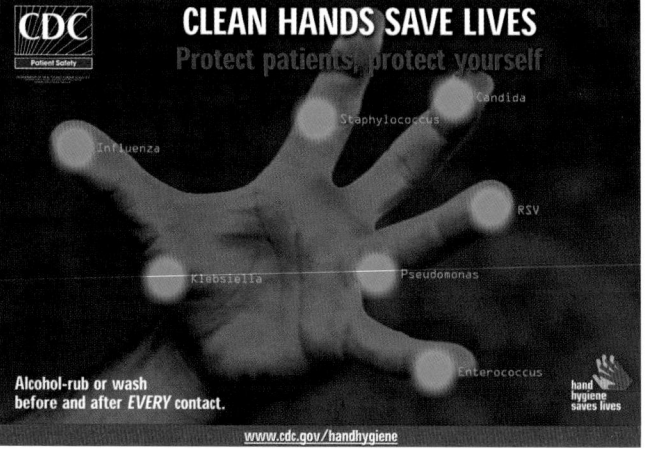

Source: Centers for Disease Control and Prevention

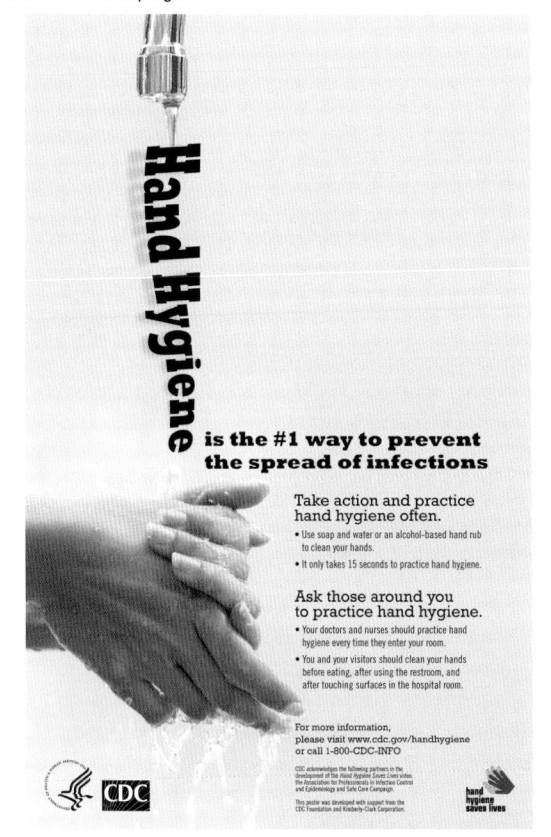

Source: Centers for Disease Control and Prevention

Healthcare workers should preferably take a shower soon *after* the completion of their work day, thereby not contaminating their own environment with potential pathogens from a clinical setting. In addition, it is vital that clean uniforms and clean underwear are worn each day.

While it may be customary for most people in Australia to shower each day, it is not necessarily viewed the same by all, including those from different cultural and ethnic backgrounds. People can choose how to conduct their own personal hygiene practices when not working. However, during day-to-day life as a healthcare worker it is crucial that daily hygiene is maintained without exception. Alongside effective handwashing routines, scrupulous personal hygiene practices are basic yet cost-effective contributions.

Personal protective equipment (PPE)

Personal protective equipment (PPE) is essential in today's healthcare setting. It provides the essential protection against the transmission of microorganisms by serving as a physical barrier. PPE can actually protect patients and healthcare workers alike.

For instance, healthcare workers are shielded from microorganisms via gloves, gowns, goggles and masks. These items largely prevent microorganisms from entering the healthcare worker's bloodstream, eyes, mouth or non-intact skin. Similarly, the patient is also protected via these same items in similar ways (see **Figure 4.6**).

While it is important that the employer provides the PPE, it is also a legal requirement that the healthcare worker uses it not only correctly but also at the correct times. This is in direct accordance with the **Workplace Health and Safety Act 2011**. Furthermore, the NHMRC have further regulated the use of PPE by stipulating that the equipment must also comply with the prescribed national Australian and New Zealand quality standards.

FIGURE 4.6 PPE protects both patients and healthcare workers

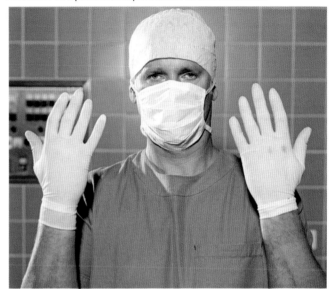

Source: Janni Chavakis/Corbis

Therefore, this begs the question: when is it appropriate to use PPE and how is this decision reached? While all healthcare settings will have their own policies and procedures pertaining to infection control practices, there are also some universal risk assessments that should be considered prior to undertaking any task. Refer to the example box *Conducting a risk assessment* on page 66 to consider the types of questions that must be posed prior to performing a clinical task.

EXAMPLE

Conducting a risk assessment

When conducting a risk assessment for a procedure, you should consider the following questions:

- What is the likelihood of transmission of microorganisms while performing this task?
- How invasive is this procedure?
- What types of bodily fluids are likely to be encountered?
- Does the patient have a known transmissible disease?
- What is the most likely route of transmission for the microorganism?

- Which items of PPE will best protect the most vulnerable sites?

Once these questions have been explored and the correct PPE is chosen for the particular task, it is then a matter of also understanding when it needs to be replaced, such as once obviously soiled and between patient interactions.

The next section summarises the common types of PPE found in healthcare settings and Australian-recommended guidelines for use.

Ordinary gloves (non-sterile)

Gloves need to be worn whenever there is a risk of contact with bodily fluids, including compromised **skin integrity** and exposure to **mucous membranes** (e.g. mouth).

It is important that gloves are *removed as soon as the task is completed*. This is usually at the point of care taking place. It is unacceptable to continue wearing them after the episode of care as this will heighten cross-contamination within the healthcare setting.

Once gloves are removed and directly disposed of in an appropriate receptacle, it is vital that hands are immediately washed.

There are many clinical examples where gloves need to be used, including:

- showering or bed-bathing a patient
- cleaning a patient's teeth or dentures
- providing perineal care to those who are incontinent of either urine or faeces, or both
- emptying receptacles that contain patient's bodily fluids (e.g. indwelling catheter bag [IDC])
- performing a **venepuncture** (blood taking)
- when disposing of any waste that accrues from any of the listed tasks.

Plastic aprons and waterproof or impervious gowns

Plastic, non-sterile aprons (usually white in appearance) are for general use in many healthcare settings where there is potential for small splashes of bodily fluids. The plastic apron will ensure that the healthcare worker's uniform is guarded against the transfer of microorganisms in general care circumstances.

Impervious (or waterproof) gowns can be either sterile or non-sterile, depending on the nature of the task to be undertaken. These gowns are chosen in preference to the plastic apron when there is a greater chance of larger splashes of bodily fluids. In other words, this is the gown of choice for more invasive and specialised procedures.

There are various clinical examples where aprons or impervious gowns need to be used, including:

- perineal care of patients who are incontinent of urine, faeces or both
- when a patient is under contact precautions to limit the contamination of the uniform and thus decrease the likelihood of the infectious transmission process
- in a surgical setting such as theatre
- in invasive procedures

- when assisting to stop a patient from dying from a major bleed
- where heightened contact precautions are required, such as when caring for someone who has scabies or patients experiencing profuse vomiting or diarrhoea.

Masks

Surgical masks are frequently used as part of standard precautions when there is likelihood of bodily fluids from a patient entering the healthcare worker's mouth or nose. In this instance, the surgical mask is used to protect the worker, not the patient.

Similarly, surgical masks may also be used when droplet precautions are in place in an effort to protect the worker.

A more specialised type of mask, called a P2 or N95 mask, has highly advanced filtering functions, superior to that of the surgical mask.

Masks may be used:

- when emptying receptacles that may contain bodily fluids such as wound drains
- with a patient with **tuberculosis (TB)** who requires droplet precautions and therefore masks would routinely be worn during all patient care
- for airborne precautions, when the P2 or N95 would be used
- during episodes of care that are considered to be at high risk for healthcare worker contamination (e.g. bronchoscopy [examination of the lungs]).

Goggles or face shields

Goggles are often used as part of standard precautions where there is a risk of bodily fluids contaminating the healthcare worker's eyes.

Face shields provide superior protection from contamination than do goggles as they have the ability to safeguard the entire face, including eyes, mouth, nose and skin.

Goggles and face shields may be used:

- when performing oral suctioning or emptying receptacles containing bodily fluids such as a suction container or IDC
- when caring for a patient who is experiencing profuse vomiting
- for more invasive procedures and where is there is a greater chance of bodily fluid splashes (e.g. in surgery) when face shields would be used in preference to goggles.

TIP BOX

Cleaning goggles and masks
Some goggles and masks are reusable and therefore must be cleaned after use. Interestingly, the front of the item is considered contaminated but the back of it is not!

Cleaning environmental surfaces

All types of cleaning practices require the use of PPE in order to protect the healthcare worker.

Broadly speaking, cleaning tasks can be separated into two distinct classifications. The first group consists of low-risk areas that are not touched by hands on a regular basis, such as floors and walls. The second group includes high-risk areas that are frequently touched by hands; for example, any patient contact regions such as beds, tables, lockers and bathrooms.

The exception to this is when it has already been established that there is a presence of pathogenic organisms. In this instance, 'normal' cleaning schedules would be heightened to account for the increased risk of transmission.

Routine cleaning

Routine cleaning is conducted daily and whenever there is a particular need, such as a spill of any nature. The main aim of cleaning is to remove surface dust that mostly consists of dead skin cells from the patients who are residing in that area. Many patients are hospitalised either because they themselves are in a compromised state or because they may harbor pathogenic microorganisms and therefore create the potential for transmission of infection.

Understandably, it is crucial that routine cleaning schedules remove this surface dust and associated particles. This is especially important in direct patient zones and where clinical procedures may be undertaken. For example, the patient's mobile bedside table that usually accommodates meals may also be used to place down wash bowls or dressings prior to use. Therefore, it is critical that these types of patient items are routinely cleaned, especially as it has a dual function.

Cleaning schedule

Although time-consuming, it is not difficult to achieve a clean environment as part of a routine cleaning schedule. Generally, all that is required is a mild detergent with warm water, facilitated by a clean cloth. This is done on a daily basis as a routine practice, but should also be conducted prior to and after each different episode of use, as well as when visibly soiled. This may include the use of disinfectants if appropriate.

In a healthcare setting that predominantly operates on a daytime schedule, such as a health clinic, these cleaning procedures would also be conducted at the beginning of the day, the completion of the day and in between each use. See the example on this page for more information.

Although it may seem like commonsense, it is important to remember that any damp cleaning procedure must also be

---

EXAMPLE

Cleaning chairs and tables

Chairs and tables in a clinic should be cleaned prior to and after use. The same routine should be conducted again if the chair or table is used for a procedure.

Chairs and tables should be routinely cleaned at the end of each working day.

---

followed by drying the item as well. When effective cleaning routines are followed, as previously described, it promotes a consistent reduction in environmental contamination.

When conducting all cleaning procedures, it is prudent to assess the quality of the surface. Any rips, breaks or compromises in surfaces offer an excellent breeding ground for microorganisms to flourish even if only because the compromised areas increase the body surface of the item. In instances where surface covers are impaired, it is important these are reported to the appropriate personnel so that replacement can be organised. This may sound like a trivial concept but all efforts to improve infection control will achieve improved outcomes. Lastly, it is equally important from a safety perspective that cleaning products are stored correctly and cleaning equipment is inspected regularly for signs of deterioration (see **Figure 4.7** on page 70).

Storage of cleaning products also requires a special log to be kept and maintained. This will itemise the type of product alongside the particular storage requirements; for example, sodium hypochlorite (commonly known as bleach) must be locked

FIGURE 4.7 Cleaning products must be stored correctly

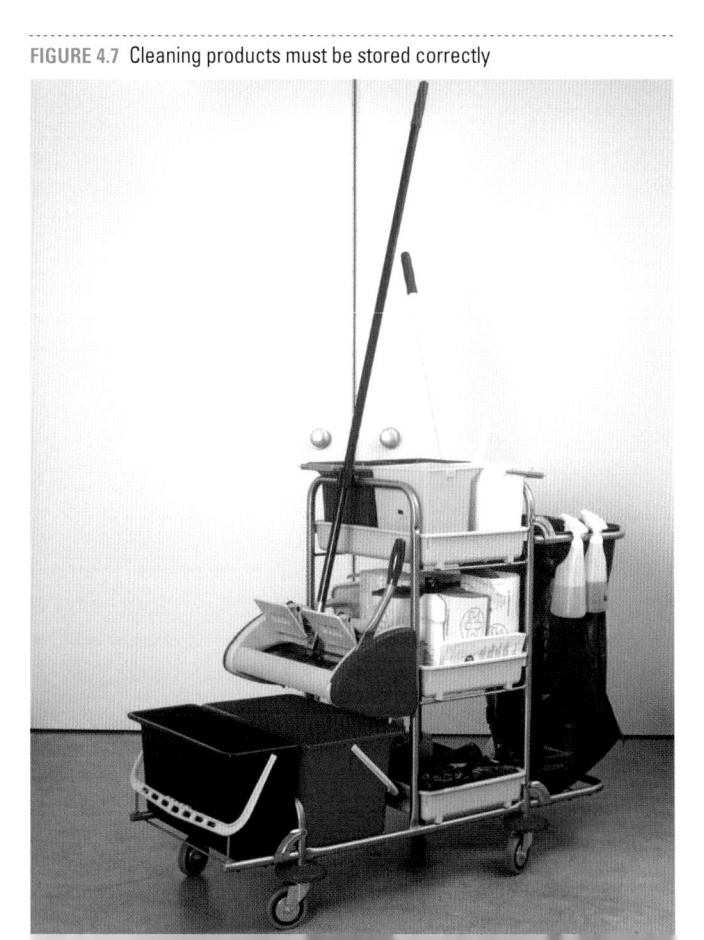

in an area whereby access is limited, mainly to the cleaning staff. There are also certain documents that accompany these guidelines to ensure that there is a written record of safe storage practices. This is called a **material safety data sheet** (MSDS) and provides information on the properties of hazardous substances (such as bleach), how they need to be stored and the impacts on health and safety within the healthcare setting.

Likewise, it is the user's responsibility to ensure that all equipment used in cleaning procedures is in good working order. It is important to inspect equipment and replace as necessary.

Sharps handling and disposal techniques

A sharp is considered to be anything that contains a needle, such as a lancet used to take blood sugar levels or a syringe and needle used for injections. Healthcare workers in various roles will potentially be required to use, handle and dispose of such sharps.

The inherent risks associated with the use of sharps include the contamination of the healthcare worker with a patient's bodily fluids, especially blood. An accidental puncture from a used sharp (commonly known as a **needle stick injury**) can adversely affect the healthcare worker, including the risk of transmission of HIV, hepatitis B and hepatitis C.

The primary aim in the management of sharps is to eliminate or reduce the risk of this possibility (see **Figure 4.8**). Many

FIGURE 4.8 Disposing of a syringe

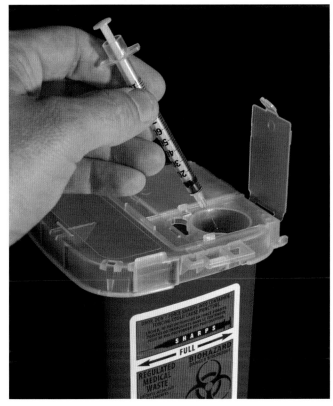

Source: sshepard/iStockphoto

FIGURE 4.9 Retractable needle

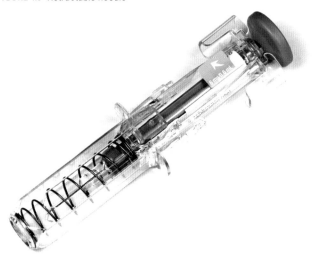

Source: ribeiroantonio/Shutterstock

healthcare settings have invested in retractable or needleless devices so as to drastically reduce or even eliminate the risk of sharps injuries (see **Figure 4.9**).

Table 4.3 on page 72 shows common risk reduction strategies for the prevention of needle stick injuries, both while handling and disposing of sharps.

TABLE 4.3 Risk reduction strategies in the prevention of needle stick injuries

Handling of sharps	Disposing of sharps
• Never recap used needles due to the potential of receiving a needle stick injury. • Eliminate or reduce passing the sharp from hand to hand. • Use of gloves is highly recommended with handling sharps, even if just for protection from accidental blood spills from patient to healthcare worker. • Maintain communication with other team members, particularly when moving the sharp from area to area.	• Never separate or remove the actual sharp from its accompanying item; for example, do not remove the needle from a syringe and then dispose of the needle. The act of removing the needle actually increases the chance of the healthcare worker receiving a needle stick injury. Leave the complete unit intact and dispose of as is. • Always use an Australian approved sharps container bearing the official code information of AS4031 or AS/NZ4261. This will ensure that the sharps bin complies with puncture proof requirements. • Never fill the sharps container above the recommended 'full' indicator. Once 'full', ensure that the lid is secured tightly and further strengthened with reinforcing tape or similar. • Ensure safe placement of sharps containers so that they cannot be accidentally knocked over, potentially causing multiple sharps injuries. It is best practice that sharps containers are mounted to a wall in some fashion; many healthcare settings fasten specific brackets to the walls for the accommodation of sharps bins. • Keep out of reach of children and also those who may be cognitively impaired.

TIP BOX

Sharp disposal
The person who has generated the sharp is ultimately responsible for its disposal!

Ensuring sterility of instruments

The concept of equipment and instrument cleansing processes follows on from environmental cleaning and it is extremely important that it is completed effectively. The level of cleaning required is dependent on the role of the instrument or piece of equipment in question. The more invasive the procedure, the greater level of cleansing required. Therefore, an instrument that probes deep inside the body will need to be sterilised (see **Figure 4.10**) as opposed to disinfected, in line with quality control practices.

Instruments and equipment fall into one of three categories: critical, semi-critical and non-critical. The NHMRC guidelines have summarised these levels, which are discussed in **Table 4.4**.

TIP BOX

Critical, semi-critical and non-critical items
Critical risk items include surgeon's instruments, semi-critical items include exploratory instruments and non-critical items include blood pressure machines.

TABLE 4.4 Risk regarding sterility

Critical risk	Instruments that fall into this category are at a high risk of transmitting pathogens if not correctly sterilised. Therefore, sterilisation for these items is imperative due to the invasive purpose that they serve.
Source: Dan Chippendale/ Getty Images	
Semi-critical risk	Instruments or pieces of equipment that fall into this category are at risk of transmitting pathogens as well but they are not used in highly invasive procedures so the risk is somewhat reduced. They are usually single-use only items or are heavily disinfected.
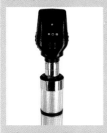 Source: bjsites/Shutterstock	
Non-critical	These items do not have invasive roles and can be either thoroughly cleansed or disinfected, but do not need sterilisation processes.
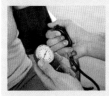 Source: Andrey_Popov/ Shutterstock	

FIGURE 4.10 Sterile articles

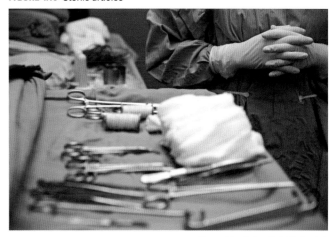

Source: Adam Radosavljevic/Shutterstock

To ensure that the item is sterile at the time of use, it is important to establish the following information:

- Is the item for an invasive procedure? If so, evidence of sterilisation is essential.
- Is the packaging of the item consistent with the standard sterilisation appearance?
- Is the packaging intact?
- Is there a date and time for when sterilisation occurred?
- Is there an expiry date of the sterilisation process for the item?

There are certain pieces of equipment that require a combination of cleansing processes due to their complex structures. For example, **endoscopes** and **bronchoscopes** are often soaked in water and concentrated detergent prior to undergoing a chemical type of sterilisation process.

In most cases, these specialised processes require specific training by a relevant organisation. In the example above, most healthcare workers would be trained to clean endoscopes or bronchoscopes in accordance with the guidelines outlined by the Gastroenterological Society of Australia (GESA) as well as the Gastroenterological Nurses College of Australia (GENCA).

SUMMARY

- Infection control guidelines in healthcare settings are crucial to infection transmission and prevention.
- Effective hand hygiene practices must be implemented.
- Sound personal hygiene practices must be adhered to.
- Ensure that PPE is used correctly when indicated.
- It is important to remember the significance of both routine and specialised cleaning practices, as guided by standard and transmission-based precautions.
- Safe sharps handling and disposal techniques are vital in the prevention of needle stick injuries.
- An equally important role of the healthcare worker is to ensure the sterility of items at the time of use. This includes instruments used in surgery which are considered a critical risk for infection transmission.

1 List 10 practices that would be included in a healthcare facility's infection control policies and procedures.

2 In the table below, outline the differences and similarities between standard and transmission-based precautions.

Type of precaution	Differences	Similarities
Standard precautions		
Transmission-based precautions		

3 Complete this sentence: _____ _____ is the single most effective infection control measure that a healthcare worker can implement.

4 In accordance with WHO guidelines, how long should each handwashing practice take in duration?
   a Social
   b Clinical
   c Surgical

5 How frequently should routine cleaning be conducted in a healthcare setting?

6 What cleaning agent is primarily used in routine cleaning of a healthcare setting?

7 Whose responsibility is it to safely dispose of a sharp?

8 State three risk reduction strategies to prevent a needle stick injury from occurring.

9 List the three risk categories for the cleansing of medical equipment and surgical instruments.

10 Which category of risk would a surgeon's scalpel fall into and why?

5 CULTURAL CONSIDERATIONS IN AUSTRALIAN HEALTHCARE

Introduction

This chapter considers 'culture' as a determinant of healthy living. Australia has a rich cultural history, and this history begins with Indigenous Australians. Aboriginal and Torres Strait Islander people comprise over 250 language groups, and there is a lot of diversity in and between groups and places. Settlers and immigrants to Australia also bring their own cultures that add to the diversity of cultural Australia today. This chapter briefly considers some of the historical issues that have contributed to the current state of Aboriginal and Torres Strait Islander health, some of the current issues facing people from non-English-speaking countries and some ways to increase cultural proficiency when working across cultures.

Understanding cultural diversity in the workplace

There are currently 270 different ethnic groups in Australia, with over 400 languages spoken across the nation.

The cultural and linguistic diversity is not bound within the walls of households but pervades all facets of Australian life, including workplaces, healthcare settings, schools, shopping malls and sporting clubs. In order to provide holistic and **culturally competent healthcare**, staff must not only be aware of the extent of such diversity, but also have the ability to incorporate safe practices into everyday work life. The healthcare industry is a service industry and so its personnel need to have the skills and knowledge to deliver care that is culturally responsive and respectful. Outlined below are some practical examples of how cultural consideration can be incorporated into everyday practice.

Protocols shaping service delivery

- Clustering new residents to residential aged care facilities (RACF) according to their cultural or language backgrounds can make for a smoother transition for new residents. This is because as a person ages, they might prefer to use their first language; clustering of residents allows for ease of preparation of cultural foods; and visitors are likely to visit the cluster, not the relative.
- Health promotion or prevention resources, such as immunisation schedules, need to be developed in community languages as well as English. A community language is a non-English language spoken in the local community. It is important to know which language, and even which dialect of that language, is the most appropriate for the local health services.
- Some cultures have gender restrictions on healthcare provision. For example, some women might prefer to have only women healthcare providers.
- Some people might have come from traumatic backgrounds, and the symptoms of trauma might be mistaken for anger or non-compliance. Taking a health history from traumatised people needs cultural sensitivity.

Cultural competence is neither limited to acknowledging differing ethnic groups, nor is it limited to languages other than English. The concepts of **cultural safety** and competence penetrate more deeply and require more attention than can be given in this context. However, in this section cultural competence will include the following principles for practice:

- Appropriate knowledge and skills are needed in order to deliver effective care in situations implicating **cultural diversity**.
- Responsive behaviours, attitudes and organisational support are required to enable a healthcare system that works effectively in cross-cultural situations.
- Effectual cultural competence enables the healthcare setting to improve health and wellbeing by incorporating cultural practices into the delivery care.

Developing personal cultural proficiency requires a lifelong learning approach to cultural competence. It is not enough to know the cultural origins of health service users. Healthcare providers need to develop cultural humility and be able to demonstrate respect for all Australians, regardless of culture or language. Some ways to increase personal cultural proficiency when working across cultures include:

- recognising that not all people moving to Australia have had the opportunity to learn English, and might need interpreter services
- understanding that being unwell might mean that some people prefer to use their community language; this might also be a side effect of ageing

- recognising that having difference in cultural practices or personal habits might be common in that culture
- retaining personal cultural humility (or being aware that no one culture is 'better' than any other), listening generously and being willing to learn, which are the most reliable ways to stay 'safe' when working across cultures.

Historical issues affecting the health of Aboriginal and Torres Strait Islander people

Aboriginal and Torres Strait Islander people have lived in Australia for at least 40 000 years, and are the oldest living cultures on earth. Before colonisation, Aboriginal and Torres Strait Islander people had healthy lifestyles. This included few infectious diseases due to living in small family-based groups with fewer people to maintain endemic diseases, such as measles or mumps.

Colonisation of Australia by settlers brought a rapid, devastating change to the health of Indigenous Australians. Across Australia, Aboriginal and Torres Strait Islander people were massacred, had their land removed and were forced to relocate to new areas; many became sick and died from introduced diseases such as smallpox. Government policies and practices saw children removed for being 'half-caste' (a very offensive term), couples required permission to marry, Aboriginal and Torres Strait Islander people were not allowed to work for government agencies and were expected to work for less money than non-Indigenous people.

Being excluded from settler society and no longer having access to the resources of their homelands meant that the Aboriginal and Torres Strait Islander population went from over 500 000 in 1788 to about 60 000 people in 1940, and Indigenous Australians were consigned to the fringes of society. These government policies and society's behaviours caused Aboriginal and Torres Strait Islander people to become poor and sick. Aboriginal and Torres Strait Islander people are still among the poorest, sickest people in Australia.

The social determinants of health and Aboriginal and Torres Strait Islander people

The recent history of Australia, including colonisation, has resulted in conditions that have led to poor health outcomes for Aboriginal and Torres Strait Islander people. These are called the **social determinants** of health. The World Health Organization (WHO) defines the social determinants of health as:

> ... the circumstances in which people are born, grow up, live, work and age, and the systems put in place to deal with illness. These circumstances are in turn shaped by a wider set of forces: economics, social policies, and politics.
>
> World Health Organization (2008)

The WHO determinants of health can be broadly considered under three headings: social and economic development, physical environment and a person's individual characteristics and behaviours. These three categories overlap and influence each other. Using the WHO's definition demonstrates that individuals do not have a lot of control over their health determinants, as each determinant affects the others (see **Figure 5.1**).

For example, if a person is born into poverty and is socially excluded because of their culture (social environment), then they are likely to live in over-crowded, substandard housing (physical environment), develop depression due to hopelessness and perhaps take to drinking alcohol (personal behaviours). Aboriginal and Torres Strait Islander people suffer 'deep disadvantage' from the determinants of health. It is the chronic, constant disadvantage Aboriginal and Torres Strait Islander people experience today that explains much of their poor health.

FIGURE 5.1 The WHO social determinants of health factors

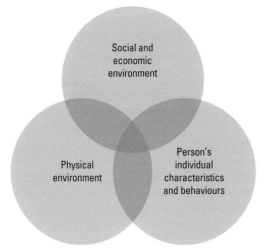

Source: Adapted from World Health Organization (n.d.). 'The determinants of health'. *Health Impact Assessment (HIA)*. http://www.who.int/hia/evidence/doh/en/

Contemporary issues in Aboriginal and Torres Strait Islander people's health

Health issues affecting Aboriginal and Torres Strait Islander people don't just carry a burden of **mortality**; they are also a great source of **morbidity**, or ongoing illness. The Commonwealth Government of Australia releases a bi-annual report called *Overcoming Indigenous Disadvantage* to report on the wellbeing of Indigenous Australians. This report considers the determinants of health, not just the health statistics. For example, the 2014 report stated the gap in life expectancy between Indigenous and non-Indigenous people has improved, and this could result from higher employment rates, fewer Indigenous people smoking tobacco and more home ownership than shown in the 2011 report.

Considering health statistics, Edith Cowan University's Health*Info*Net – a resource devoted to gathering information regarding the health of Indigenous Australians – puts together a report from various sources, including the Australian Bureau of Statistics, Commonwealth and State health departments and other non-government sources. The 2013 Overview Report stated that the main cause of hospitalisation for Aboriginal and Torres Strait Islander people between 2010 and 2012 was kidney disease, including the need for dialysis. Renal disease in Aboriginal and Torres Strait Islander people is often a result of chronic skin diseases and infections in childhood, which occur because of overcrowding, poverty and generations of exclusion from paid employment. This is part of the cycle of disadvantage that continues in Aboriginal and Torres Strait Islander communities today.

According to the Australian Indigenous Health*Info*Net report (2014), there are many competing health issues pertaining to Aboriginal and Torres Strait Islander people. Although there is insufficient time to explore these in depth, it is important to gain an understanding of the types of particular health issues that are of greatest concern in Aboriginal and Torres Strait Islander populations. These are illustrated in **Table 5.1**.

TABLE 5.1 Contemporary issues in Aboriginal and Torres Strait Islander health

Disease or condition	Rates (comparison between Indigenous and non-Indigenous)	Mortality (death rate from this condition)
Cardiovascular disease (CVD)	CVD rates are approximately twice as high in the Indigenous Australian populations than in non-Indigenous people	More than 25% of deaths were from CVD. CVD was the greatest cause of death for Indigenous Australians
Cancer	Indigenous Australians are 1.5 times more likely to receive a fatal cancer diagnosis than non-Indigenous people	Cancer was the second greatest cause of death in this time frame
Diabetes	Effects of diabetes are more than three times higher in Indigenous populations than in non-Indigenous	Indigenous Australians die of diabetes at seven times the rate of other Australians
Social and emotional wellbeing deficit	Indigenous Australians were almost three times more likely to report high or very high levels of psychological distress	Nearly twice the mortality rate compared to non-Indigenous counterparts and this did not include suicide
Kidney disease	Indigenous Australians were seven times more likely to experience kidney disease	Indigenous Australians were four times more likely to die from kidney-related disease
Accidents/injuries	Indigenous Australians were twice as likely to experience injuries from accidents than non-Indigenous people	Injuries from accidents (largely traffic related) were the third most common cause of death
Respiratory disease	Indigenous Australians were almost three times more likely to be admitted to hospital due to respiratory conditions	Indigenous people died from respiratory disease and complications twice as often as non-Indigenous

Disease or condition	Rates (comparison between Indigenous and non-Indigenous)	Mortality (death rate from this condition)
Eye conditions	Eye conditions were almost three times more likely to occur in Indigenous populations, while blindness was at least six times more likely	N/A
Ear conditions	Just over 1 in 10 Indigenous Australians are either partially or completely deaf Hospitalisation from ear disease was 1.3 times higher in Indigenous populations	N/A
Oral health conditions	Indigenous Australians had more than double the oral cavities and higher rates of gingivitis than non-Indigenous populations	N/A
Communicable diseases (also known as infectious diseases)	Tuberculosis (TB) rates were 11 times higher in Indigenous populations Influenza type B rates were 20 times high in Indigenous populations Sexually transmitted infections (STIs) were up to 64 times higher in Indigenous populations	Unfortunately this study did not provide information regarding mortality rates for any communicable diseases N/A

Source: Adapted from Australian Indigenous Health*Info*Net (2014). Summary of Australian Indigenous Health, 2013. http://www.healthinfonet.ecu.edu.au/health-facts/summary

Communicable diseases in Aboriginal and Torres Strait Islander communities

Contrary to popular opinion, 75 per cent of Aboriginal and Torres Strait Islander people live in urban or metropolitan areas, and the majority live in NSW. There is a lot of difference between communities but there is a lot in common as well. The commonalities are often because of the pressures of the determinants of health. Infectious, or communicable, diseases contribute to the burden of disease experienced by Aboriginal and Torres Strait Islander communities.

Tables 5.1 and 5.2 indicate that some communicable diseases can be linked to the determinants of health. Reducing the rates of these diseases requires health professionals to think about the way in which Aboriginal and Torres Strait Islander people might live, what resources they have and even what beliefs about diseases some people might have.

Immunisation in Aboriginal and Torres Strait Islander communities

One of the greatest public health successes is the on-going immunisation program in Aboriginal and Torres Strait Islander communities. For

TABLE 5.2 Infectious and communicable diseases experienced in Aboriginal and Torres Strait Islander communities

Disease	Transmission	Health determinants
Tuberculosis (TB)	Droplet infection	Overcrowded houses, poverty, smoking, alcohol abuse, malnutrition, diabetes and kidney disease
Hepatitis (A, B, C)	Ingestion of virus	Poor housing, poor access to water, poor knowledge of disease process
Hepatitis C	Bloodborne virus	Poor social and emotional wellbeing (leads to IV drug use)
Haemophilus influenzae type B (HIB)	Droplet infection	Poverty, overcrowding, poor nutrition, chronic illness
Pneumococcal disease	Droplet infection	Age, diabetes, chronic diseases, immunocompromised people, smoking, alcohol abuse
Meningococcal disease	Droplet infection	Overcrowding, being exposed to smoking
Sexually transmitted diseases	Contact with infected person	Poverty, poor education, risk-taking behaviours associated with hopelessness
HIV/AIDS	Viral infection	Poverty, risky behaviours
Skin diseases		Overcrowding, poverty, poor environment (no water)

example, approximately 92 per cent of Aboriginal and Torres Strait Islander children were fully immunised in 2013, representing a 10 per cent increase since 2003. Vaccinations in older Aboriginal and Torres Strait Islander people have offered protection against chest infections and have helped produce increased community health.

Cross-cultural belief systems

Not all Aboriginal and Torres Strait Islander people have identical beliefs and protocols, so it is necessary to always check. Some Aboriginal and Torres Strait Islander people believe they are sick because of 'wrong-way' business, where they have done 'something wrong' according to their personal beliefs. Other Aboriginal and Torres Strait Islander people might believe they have ingested something (like a worm) that is causing the disease (even chest infections).

Because people have different health belief systems, they will have different ideas on disease management. This might mean that a health professional needs to include cultural considerations in the health assessment and, while still being culturally respectful, be able to create a health management plan based on evidence, but without alienating the patient. When a person feels their beliefs have been mocked or even misunderstood, they will probably be non-compliant with their health management plan. Non-compliance in regard to communicable diseases affects more than one person, so it is important for the health of the community that treatment is continued until medical professionals advise otherwise.

Access and equity considerations

Access and equity issues are highly topical for all Australians. For example, women living in rural Australia are more likely to have radical mastectomies as treatment for breast cancer because they do not have access to the health options of women living in major cities. It is the same for Aboriginal and Torres Strait Islander people living in rural and remote areas of Australia, where the access is poor, and the services are unreliable or not culturally appropriate.

Some Aboriginal and Torres Strait Islander people are unable to afford the cost of travel to metropolitan areas to access some services, such as dialysis, and also may not be confident in speaking English. Travelling away from one's homeland is financially expensive and can be a lonely experience, and so an Aboriginal or Torres Strait Islander person will often present to a healthcare provider with a greater degree of illness and at a later stage in a disease or condition as their resources to access the healthcare, both personal and material, are hard to muster.

The history of hospitalisation for Aboriginal and Torres Strait Islander people is fraught with institutionalised racism. When an organisation has differential access to services or opportunities, it is said to have institutionalised racism. For example, in the past Aboriginal and Torres Strait Islander mothers could go to hospital for childbirth, but their babies would be 'taken away'. Aboriginal and Torres Strait Islander people would be reluctant to go to hospital for these reasons, and they also might feel discriminated against in such areas as emergency departments. Racism, where a person is treated poorly due to their ethnicity, is a major reason for the poor mental health of Aboriginal and Torres Strait Islander people.

These types of constraints are evidenced by a distinct lack of healthcare service utilisation. Furthermore, due to the lack of culturally appropriate services available, many Aboriginal and Torres Strait Islander people do not participate in screening and prevention programs, meaning that they often present with symptoms consistent with an advanced diagnosis. This in itself will produce poorer health outcomes or projected **prognoses**, but may also mean that the Aboriginal or Torres Strait Islander person could be less likely to accept offers of treatment if a disease process is already well advanced.

The following example highlights how access to culturally appropriate care can be facilitated and shows that it is possible for non-Indigenous workers to liaise appropriately with Aboriginal and Torres Strait Islander people in order to provide culturally competently care.

EXAMPLE

Facilitating culturally appropriate care

The example below, drawn from Juli Coffin's work, is a protocol between midwives and an Aboriginal community. It indicates how protocols establish patterns of behaviour that meet the specific community needs and their internal processes for making decisions.

After talking with the Aboriginal health worker, midwives discovered that the older ladies were the ones to speak to in relation to the young pregnant women. Now whenever anything with the young Mums arises there is an established point of contact to the older women first – thus an assurance is created for cultural security. Community leaders are made aware of the situation and are involved. Community participation can then be progressed beyond just 'involvement'. Communities become partners in an equitable, culturally secure provision of service, This is the pathway to cultural security.

Source: Australian Human Rights Commission (2011). 'Chapter 4: Cultural safety and security: Tools to address lateral violence'. *Social Justice Report 2011*. https://www.humanrights.gov.au/publications/chapter-4-cultural-safety-and-security-tools-address-lateral-violence-social-justice

Remember, not all Aboriginal and Torres Strait Islander communities share protocols, so the healthcare provider needs to 'check it out' first.

The questions below can help you assess the willingness of a health organisation to contribute to closing the gap in Aboriginal and Torres Strait Islander health disadvantage.

To determine the cultural proficiency of a healthcare service, ask the following:

- Are all staff trained and credentialed in cultural proficiency (e.g. have they had training; are there cultural mentors for non-Indigenous staff)?
- Would Aboriginal and Torres Strait Islander people feel welcome when they use the service (e.g. are there Indigenous-specific health posters, information pamphlets, and Aboriginal or Torres Strait Islander staff working at the service)?
- Are the services within the financial reach of Aboriginal and Torres Strait Islander clients (e.g. is there travel assistance available; are prescriptions affordable)?

- Does the health service measure attendance, use of services and satisfaction rates by Aboriginal and Torres Strait Islander people?
- Does the service have an Elder or Health Liaison Officer to assist Aboriginal and Torres Strait Islander people with health services?

If any of the answers are no, it would be worth raising this with your supervisor and seeing if you can work together to improve the healthcare environment you are working in.

EXAMPLE

Personal cultural proficiency

As an enrolled nurse, you also have a responsibility to make your patients feel comfortable through your own cultural awareness. The short checklist below provides examples for clinicians to consider personal cultural proficiency.

- Do you ensure your communication is understood by the healthcare recipient?
- Are your values more important than the healthcare recipient? (If they are, there is a risk of institutionalised racism.)
- Do you recognise that 'family' is defined differently across cultures?
- Do you realise that beliefs about some illnesses, such as mental illness, are culturally based?
- Do you accept and realise that different cultures have different ideas about food, hygiene practices and responses to illnesses?

This is just a quick checklist – there are many other salient points to consider when working across cultures. Use the local health workers to get the best fit for the communities being served by the health organisation.

Read the case study below to understand how effectively connecting with Aboriginal and Torres Strait Islander cultures can have a cumulative effect, directly affecting the social determinants of health.

CASE STUDY

Influenza in Indigenous communities

Influenza is a respiratory tract infection that is highly contagious. Every year about five to 10 per cent of Australians catch 'the flu', often suffering more than one episode. Indigenous people are at a significantly higher risk of catching influenza, and during 2009 were more likely to need admission to hospital from influenza and more likely to die than non-Indigenous people.

Indigenous Australians living in remote communities have a higher risk of catching influenza because of increased exposure to the virus, and greater risk of getting sick due to the complications and consequences of the virus. The increased risk is due to the socioeconomic and cultural determinants of health, such as over-crowding. When large families live together, it increases the transmission of the influenza virus. Other risk factors include remote communities having poor road access in tropical seasons; small, young populations (400–500

residents, more than half of which are under 30); and less access to a doctor.

Indigenous Australians might have different health-seeking behaviours, either because they have normalised being sick or due to institutionalised racism in health services. Other non-Indigenous specific risk factors include smoking and/or living in a house with smokers, and not being vaccinated against influenza.

Learning from the 2009 influenza pandemic, public health authorities now recognise the need to vaccinate as many people in the community that qualify, and to vaccinate early in the 'flu' season. Other social determinants of health, such as access to clean water, availability of fresh nutritious food and affordability of hygiene and cleaning products all contribute to the increased risk of contracting influenza.

Questions

1 Why does overcrowding increase the transmission of influenza?

2 In the 2009 pandemic, smokers and non-smokers caught influenza at the same rate. Why?

3 To what degree do you think the social determinants of health affect the rate of people catching influenza?

Source: Adapted from Chidgzey, P. J., Davis, S., Williams, P. & Reeve, C. (2015). An outbreak of influenza A (H1N1) virus in a remote Aboriginal community post-pandemic: implications for pandemic planning and health service policy. *Australian and New Zealand Journal of Public Health*, 39(1), 15–20.

TIP BOX

Respectful communication with Elders

Referring to an Elder or leader as Aunty or Uncle may not be appropriate for an outsider unless a strong relationship has been established, or unless you have asked the Aunty or Elder what they would prefer to be called.

Enhancing access and equity

The following discussion will highlight certain practice tips that have been proven to enhance concepts of access and equity in many healthcare settings.

Local knowledge

Healthcare services should be encouraged to familiarise themselves with the cultural backgrounds of where they work. This may include viewing local maps, and getting to know the Indigenous language groups and general history of the area.

Community engagement

It can be useful to research local Aboriginal and Torres Strait Islander organisations and create a working relationship with them. If approached with a transparent intention, most local Aboriginal Land Councils are pleased to provide support including the provision of resources such as maps. Another way to engage the community is to ask Aboriginal and Torres Strait Islander staff to conduct education sessions about the history of their own region.

A clear advantage of establishing community advisory groups is the increased likelihood of developing culturally relevant and sensitive service delivery.

Family and gender issues

Be aware and respectful of relevant family and kinship structures when working with Aboriginal and Torres Strait Islander people. This often means including the extended family in important meetings and decision-making processes. Show respect by ensuring that Elders and leaders in the community are involved in the decision-making processes.

If organising meetings with community members, discuss whether or not the topic of conversation is suitable for everyone or if the issue of **men's and women's business** will apply. It may require another staff member to facilitate another session so that separate sessions for women and men are offered. Where possible, it is preferable for men to speak to men and for women to speak to women, especially in circumstances where you are not known by the person or community. There may be times when non-Indigenous people may be asked to leave the room during Aboriginal and Torres Strait Islander Men's or Women's Business. It is important not to take offence to this as it indicates that sensitive or gender-specific issues will be discussed.

Sorry business

Respect cultural values and protocols for Aboriginal and Torres Strait Islander people participating in **sorry business**. Aboriginal and Torres Strait Islander people embrace sorry business by allowing a dedicated grieving time as a sign of respect for the person who has passed away. During this time, there is no expectation of work commitments or similar. Non-Indigenous people can comply with this cultural norm by specifically not requesting meetings or work-related activities for a period of two weeks or as advised by the community. Furthermore, it is important to avoid displaying or broadcasting images of deceased people. If it is important to do so, make sure that you have permission from the person's family and/or community and include a relevant disclaimer.

Communication etiquette

Respect, acknowledge, actively listen and respond to the needs of Aboriginal and Torres Strait Islander people and communities in a culturally appropriate manner. For example, some Aboriginal and Torres Strait Islander people or community groups may think it is inappropriate for a non-Indigenous person to refer to them by their state name (e.g. Koori, Murri). However, if you establish a good rapport with them, they will appreciate the terminology once you have been given permission to use it. Consult with Aboriginal and Torres Strait Islander staff within the department or other government departments if you are unsure of etiquette requirements.

Communicate with sensitivity

When working in the healthcare environment it is important to be sensitive in your approach. You should:

- respect the use of silence and don't mistake it for misunderstanding a topic or issue
- always wait your turn to speak

- speak clearly and as loud as necessary, but do not shout
- sensitively offer assistance with reading and writing if it is required
- be mindful of potential language barriers
- use clear, uncomplicated language; do not use jargon.

Do not continually ask a person to repeat themselves if it is difficult to understand them, especially in front of a large group.

Show cultural understanding

When dealing with Aboriginal and Torres Strait Islander people in a healthcare setting, avoid making assumptions. For example, you should note the following:

- While some people from an Aboriginal and Torres Strait Islander background will avoid eye contact as a sign of respect, it is important to remember that this is not always the case and is dependent on an individual's tradition.
- Different words might have different meanings in different communities.
- Swear words may be a part of normal conversation.
- The definition of Aboriginality is a person must have Aboriginal parentage; must identify as an Aboriginal person; and must be accepted by the Aboriginal community as an Aboriginal person. However, the words 'Aboriginal' or 'Indigenous' are used in different places across Australia, and areas will have their own preference for which word to use. Always check the local use of these terms.
- Indigenous identity – health service providers must ask health service users if they identify as Aboriginal and/or Torres Strait Islanders in order to collect data to provide appropriate services.

It is important to ask and not to assume by one's appearance, as Aboriginal and Torres Strait Islander people come in all appearances and it is impossible to judge 'Aboriginality'.

- When you are directly referring to Torres Strait Islander people, use the term 'Torres Strait Islander' or 'Torres Strait Islander person'.
- It is important to use capital first letters for Aboriginal, Torres Strait Islander and Indigenous in the same way as the use of the capital A in Australia.

Communicate appropriately with a crowd

When addressing a group, it is important to:

- acknowledge land and original custodians when addressing a group of Aboriginal and Torres Strait Islander people
- organise official 'Welcome to Country' speeches for large forums, conferences and gatherings.

TIP BOX

Walking on eggshells

One of the most common fears of non-Indigenous people working with Aboriginal and Torres Strait Islander people is that they will 'make a mistake' and cause offence. However, we all make mistakes, and the best remedy is to apologise for any offence caused and then move forward. Develop trust in your healthcare service users by being trustworthy and trusting. Working with Aboriginal and Torres Strait Islander people is both challenging and rewarding.

SUMMARY

- It is vital to have an understanding of cultural diversity in healthcare settings in order provide holistic and culturally-appropriate care
- There are many historical issues that have caused health disparities for Aboriginal and Torres Strait Islander people.
- Particular health issues relating to the Aboriginal and Torres Strait Islander populations include cardiovascular disease, cancer, diabetes, social and emotional wellbeing deficits, kidney disease, accidents/injuries, eye conditions, ear conditions, respiratory disease, oral health conditions and communicable diseases.
- Access and equity issues remain persistent barriers to improving the health of Australia's Aboriginal and Torres Strait Islander people. Many healthcare settings are designed for non-Indigenous Australians.
- The majority of Aboriginal and Torres Strait Islander people live in urban settings, while those in remote areas often have limited access to healthcare services.

REVIEW QUESTIONS

1. Where do the majority of Aboriginal and Torres Strait Islander people live?
2. Are healthcare services as easily accessible in Australia's rural and remote regions as they are in metropolitan areas?
3. In the *Summary of Australian Indigenous health 2012–2013* study, what was the leading cause of death for Australia's Aboriginal and Torres Strait Islander population?
4. What would be a culturally appropriate course of action to take if unable to clearly understand an Aboriginal or Torres Strait Islander client's speech?
5. Are there more or less Aboriginal and Torres Strait Islander people living with diabetes compared with non-Indigenous people?
6. Which form of immunisation has had a positive effect on chest infections in the Aboriginal and Torres Strait Islander community?
7. What are some of the health determinants of tuberculosis?

6 ORGANISATIONAL INFECTION CONTROL POLICIES AND PROCEDURES

Introduction

Organisational **policies** and **procedures** are paramount to the success of healthcare services' infection control objectives. Healthcare workers need to not only understand the policies and procedures of an organisation, but also have a working knowledge of circumstances that may indicate the initiation of heightened infection control measures. Similarly, all such activities are not complete until an evaluation process has been incorporated into the plan. Collectively, these measures all contribute to the ongoing quality improvement in infection control practices.

Identifying policies and procedures underpinning infection control processes

Policies, procedures, **guidelines**, **implementation standards** and **protocols** are the documents that guide healthcare workers' actions when undertaking infection control measures. **Table 6.1** provides an overview of these documents.

Below is a more rigorous examination of policies, procedures, guidelines and implementation standards. We will scrutinise their content as well as compare and contrast their similarities.

Procedures

State government health services outline generic policies and procedures, ensuring uniform consistency across the state. A procedure needs to include the purpose, scope and the actual proposed procedure relevant to the clinical issue.

TABLE 6.1 Infection control documentation

Policy	A document that prescribes the particular organisation's intent to achieve a desired outcome. Policy compliance is mandatory.
Procedure	A recommended set of practices usually presented in a sequential manner. Provision of a procedure supports consistency and an expected level of quality across an organisation, in the performance of the activity or service to be provided.
Guideline	A document that supports decision making and provides advice on best practice.
Implementation standard	A document that specifies the minimum actions required to comply with a policy. This standard will identify actions and responsibilities for staff. Implementation standard compliance is mandatory.
Protocol	A document containing specific guidelines, expected to be followed in detail. There is little scope for variation. Protocol compliance is mandatory.

TIP BOX ◐

Procedures and PPE

The use of PPE is covered in a procedure for practical application. Like most procedures, the purpose and scope is often brief and succinct for ease of use for the clinician.

The actual procedure is usually quite detailed and will include any type of circumstance. This can include anything from the appropriate use of gloves (**Figure 6.1**) through to the use of high-visibility vests. It also includes issues of non-compliance, ongoing training in the use of PPE, approved PPE items and the when, where and who of use.

FIGURE 6.1 Clinical gloves

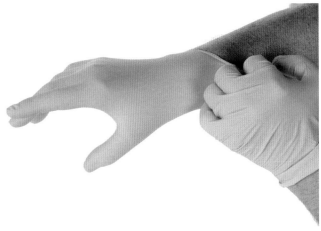

Source: Jeffrey B. Banke/Shutterstock

In addition, the procedure will include other areas for consideration such as replacement, cleaning and storage requirements. This is further supported by policies, procedures, guidelines and legislation that complement or are associated with the relevant procedure document.

Policies

A policy needs to include purpose, application, associated legislation or relevant standards (such as employee award agreements), subject and the contents of the actual policy statement. Similar to the contents of a procedure, a policy will include a short synopsis of the purpose, application and associated legislation or standards. The focus is on the content of the statement and is often divided into sections and displayed in the table of contents, as shown in the example on this page.

Guidelines

Guidelines can be less prescriptive in nature but also have common threads between them. For example, if considering the guidelines on the management of impetigo (caused by *Staphylococcus aureus*

EXAMPLE

An example of a policy 'table of contents'

Shipsey and Unnasch Community Hospital
Hand Hygiene Policy and Procedure
Table of Contents

1	Introduction
2	The underpinning elements to ensure adequate hand hygiene
3	Performing hand hygiene
3.1	Types of hand hygiene
3.1.1	Social hand wash
3.1.2	Clinical hand wash
4	Requirements to perform hand hygiene
5	The procedure for performing hand hygiene
6	Hand drying
7	Use of alcohol-based hand rub
7.1	How to use alcohol-based hand rub
7.2	Best practice points
8	Nail care
9	Hand hygiene and jewellery
10	Hand hygiene and work clothing
11	Hand care

or *Streptococcus pyogenes*) or any other types of highly infectious pathogens, there is an expectation it would include the following topics:

- Establishing diagnosis via pathology testing
- Outlining the need for isolation as relevant
- Types of precautions to be implemented; for example, contact precautions are required for the management of impetigo
- Duration of precautions
- Hand hygiene requirements and use of PPE
- Guidelines for visitors
- Cleaning requirements, including cleaning of patient equipment or devices
- Surveillance issues
- Monitoring of increases in cases
- Consideration of antimicrobial stewardship, which simply means the judicious prescribing and administering of antibiotics when clinically indicated.

Implementation standards

An implementation standard is similar to a policy and procedure in its contents. An implementation standard needs to include the:

- purpose
- scope
- supporting legislation or documents
- requirements of the guidelines.

For example, a workplace health and safety implementation standard may include risk and hazard identification, associated management processes and issues of accountability.

Contributors supporting the infection control process

Management of infection control processes does not only occur within the clinical setting. Other support services within and interacting with the healthcare environment play a large part in ensuring that infection control processes flow as they should and contribute to the overall management of infection control processes.

These may include but are not limited to:

- local public health units
- local government services
- cleaning or operational support services
- equipment cleaning, storage and management
- hazard identification and risk management
- quality system documentation and processes
- staff immunisation programs.

Local public health units

Local public health units formulate and provide specialised disease control initiatives, focused policy and procedure direction to health services, other sectors and the community. Direct procedural advice is provided for management of serious public health issues including norovirus, rotavirus, influenza viruses and tuberculosis.

Local government services

Waste management services provided by local government may be required to provide increased services in response to localised outbreaks of disease. Prompt and frequent waste disposal assists management of infection and decreases opportunity for re-infection.

Operational support services and cleaning services

Protocols and procedures exist for environmental cleaning and spills management. These protocols and work directives prescribe step-by-step best practice to effectively minimise infection risks.

Work instructions directing the appropriate use of chemicals and frequency of cleaning include specific instructions for management of and work environment cleaning related to contamination by multi-resistant organisms (Queensland Department of Health, 2014). This includes, but is not limited to, vancomycin-resistant enterococci (VRE) and *Clostridium difficile* infections.

Equipment cleaning, storage and management

Specific work instructions exist directing the use of equipment, both reusable or single-use, including storage and cleaning instructions for non-disposable equipment. Visit the CHRISP website and refer to the guidelines *Management of multi-resistant organisms*, at http://www.health.qld.gov.au/chrisp >

Management plans and guidance > Guidelines and policy framework > Management of multi-resistant organisms (MROs)

Hazard identification and risk management

'A hazard is a situation or thing that has the potential to harm a person' (Queensland Department of Health, 2014). Identifying and managing hazards and risks directly contributes to the effective management of infection control.

Quality system documentation and processes

Establishing and using quality system documentation enables recording, tracking and trending of infection control data. This data allows for the identification of areas that require improvement, formulation and implementation of improved processes and procedures, as well as evaluating the effectiveness of the improvements (Australian Commission on Safety and Quality in Health Care, 2011).

Staff immunisation programs

To help control the spread of infection, many organisations now have a Work Health and Safety policy requiring staff immunisations. Immunisations required may change with the work that staff are required to undertake in different roles. The underpinning rationale for staff immunisation programs is to offer protection from disease to both staff and clients. Granting of employment may be conditional on a staff member's agreement to undertake required immunisations (Queensland Health, 2013).

Workplace documentation

Workplace documentation is crucial not only to guide practice, but also to provide evidence of the care provided. Excellence in care can be demonstrated by following sound organisational policies and procedures, and supported by accurate and objective documentation to reflect clinical compliance.

Accessing policies and procedures

It is expected that employees will be given access and direction to policies and procedures during their scheduled orientation and once commencing employment. Once staff are given this information, they are expected to not only peruse the documentation, but also consult them as a clinical need arises.

The manner in which healthcare workers access organisational policies and procedures is largely dependent on the nature of the facility or service. Most organisations have computerised systems to accommodate written policies and procedures; however, this is not a mandatory requirement. Many smaller organisations that do not have extensive IT infrastructure will simply print the documents from a centralised computer and keep them in folders that are easily accessible to staff.

In order for the policies and procedures to be true working documents, they must be located in areas where staff are able to refer to them quickly and readily. They cannot be stored away in a locked office or similar as they simply will not be used.

Recording infection control risks and incidents

It is usual practice to record clinical observations of a client's signs of infection as well as steps undertaken to ascertain if infection is indeed present. Documenting this information is imperative to ensure it is available for all members of the multidisciplinary team to access. Continuing observations and recording of data will provide a clear clinical picture of how the infection is evolving or responding to treatment and will assist in the decision-making process guiding future interventions.

Further entry of infection details on a dedicated 'Infection log' will capture information and enable trend tracking by the healthcare facility.

Infection control risk assessment provides data to assist in a client's health management. For example, an overweight diabetic client who is about to undergo surgery requires a risk assessment, including information on glycaemic control, as this will have a direct effect on expected wound healing and associated infection risk.

Interpreting infection control records

In some healthcare institutions such as residential aged care facilities, pathology results are sometimes interpreted by nursing staff who then contact the doctor if further treatment is required. A pathology result report is shown in **Figure 6.2**. Take a moment to familiarise yourself with the format and the information presented in the report.

ACTIVITY

Reading a pathology report

Use the pathology report in **Figure 6.2** and answer the following questions.

1 What type of specimen does this pathology report provide results for?
2 From which part of the body was the specimen collected?
3 Name the antibiotic the infective organism is resistant to.
4 Name the antibiotics the infective organism is sensitive to.
5 Name the infective organism.

FIGURE 6.2 A pathology report

Pus/Wounds/Genitals/Mucopus	
Specimen	
Specimen Type:	Wound Swab
Description:	abdo
Microscopy	
Leucocytes	**not seen**
Epithelial Cells	**occasional**
No organisms seen	
Culture	
Mixed Growth Including:	
1. Staphylococcus aureus	sparse growth
Sensitivities	1
Clindamycin	S
Dicloxacillin/Cephalothin	S
Erythromycin	S
Penicillin G	R
Comment	
Isolate(s) Possible Pathogen(s)	
Requesting Doctor: Kerswell Dr DW	
End of Report	

Combining infection control information and reports

Surveillance, recording and collation of episodes of infection within a healthcare facility provide valuable information and present the opportunity to identify trends and formulate procedural improvements in clinical practice and environmental controls.

An example could be that during a norovirus outbreak in a residential aged care facility, some clients become re-infected with the disease even though they had been placed in isolation and had stringent room cleaning performed during the initial acute phase of the illness until symptoms resolved. Furthermore, a final extensive room clean was performed when a client was symptom-free. A meeting was convened with a representative from each stream of employees working in the facility in an attempt to pinpoint why some residents became re-infected while others did not.

One procedural difference was identified and clearly divided the re-infected residents from those who did not experience re-infection. During the initial phase of the outbreak within the facility, rigorous 'end of illness' room cleaning had included replacement of window curtains. When the stock of fresh window curtains became exhausted, the room cleaners were unable to replace these items. The residents who became re-infected had not had their window curtains replaced and this was ultimately found to be the factor which enabled re-infection to occur. Stock of fresh window curtains was obtained and included as an essential component of the final room cleaning procedure.

Gathering and sharing information allows for comprehensive revision and analysis of data and is an essential component in the quality improvement cycle and the provision of best practice.

Communicating the importance of policies and procedures

Infection control policies and procedures are not simply good guidelines or best practices to aspire to. Implementing these documents is an obligation in accordance with current legislation. All staff should have a working understanding of infection control policies and procedures. This includes operational staff such as cleaners, food services, laundry services, volunteer workers and pastoral care workers. To achieve this baseline, education and further support must be provided. Appropriate-level education, as well as informal discussion and supportive direction presented by registered staff, is essential for ensuring an effective infection control process and, as a result, the safety of patients. Individual conversations with each division of staff will allow for information to be presented in their familiar context. For example, the registered or enrolled nurse can discuss with pastoral care workers information and interventions tailored to address their involvement with patients.

Both the *Work Health and Safety Act 2011* and the *Public Health Act 2005* outline that employees are required to identify, minimise and manage risks associated with healthcare provision and this includes issues relating to infection control.

A breach of infection control policies and procedures could also imply a breach in the aforementioned legislation. Failure to act in accordance with the prescribed policies and procedures could result in disciplinary action or worse. In the case of an adverse clinical event, the situation will be analysed in accordance with the service's policies and procedures. This may lead to legal ramifications for the healthcare worker, including the possibility of a coroner's inquest.

Therefore, it is not only a clinical and legal requirement to abide by set policies and procedures for the sake of patient safety and organisational integrity, but it is also a safeguard for healthcare workers.

Identifying when to implement policies and procedures

Identifying events that require the prompt implementation of infection control policies and procedures is obvious once a diagnosis has been established. The example below illustrates two infection control scenarios.

EXAMPLE

Implementing infection control policies

If a patient has been diagnosed with *Staphylococcus aureus* in their wound by pathology testing, then it is a straightforward process of referring to that particular policy, procedure or guideline and implementing the appropriate infection control strategies, such as contact precautions.

However, prior to diagnosis, a healthcare worker may suspect an infection in a patient due to clinical indications. In the case where *Giardia* is suspected, the patient may present with numerous loose and offensive smelling faeces, often accompanied by abdominal pain, fatigue and, in severe cases, fever. It is the healthcare worker's responsibility to notice these signs and symptoms and instigate the collection of a faecal specimen to be tested by pathology. Prior to diagnosis the healthcare worker should act with caution and treat the patient as having an infection requiring contact precautions.

The ability to identify such events takes keen observation and assessment skills on behalf of the healthcare worker. It also requires the healthcare worker to evaluate signs and symptoms in conjunction with one another. For instance, if a patient reports three loose bowel motions, the worker needs to ask about other clinical symptomology. If there are no other accompanying signs or symptoms, then it is not necessary to isolate the patient or use contact precautions. However, it is very important that other symptomology is identified when and if it presents so that precautions can be implemented promptly if required.

CASE STUDY

When to isolate a patient

As a newly appointed healthcare worker, you have secured a position in a residential aged care facility (RACF). You are assigned to a secure unit caring for people with varying forms of dementia. You notice that one of your residents, Mary, has just had a loose and offensive bowel motion when you took her to the toilet at morning tea time. However, she is able to take herself to the toilet at times, so you ask her if she has had any other motions of a similar nature. She cannot provide a clear answer due to her cognitive impairment. You are now left wondering if this recent bowel motion was the first of its kind or if she had previously experienced other loose motions. In addition, she cannot tell you if she has any abdominal pain or fatigue. However, she has displayed behaviours such as a grimaced facial expression and is refusing food or fluids.

Questions

1   From the information provided, explain whether or not you would isolate Mary and justify your reasoning.
2   Identify two observations regarding her symptomology that contributed to your decision.
3   Based on your decision, outline the course of action you would take next.

Implementing infection control policies and procedures

Once the infection control policies and procedures have been accessed, read and understood, it is vital that they are acted upon. Preparation is an important part of the implementation process.

On any given workday, a healthcare setting is almost always a very busy environment. Therefore, sometimes employees simply do not have the time to gather equipment, PPE and other essentials necessary in the event of an infection-related incident.

It is important that all requirements for implementing infection control procedures are ready in advance and easily accessible to all staff. Many services will have dedicated boxes, cupboards or similar storing items for specific use. For instance, many facilities have outbreak kits, packed and ready to be used as and when necessary; for example, in the event of a norovirus outbreak, there should be a pre-prepared kit containing all of the items to implement contact precautions, including a copy of the procedure or policy and also appropriate signage that needs to be displayed. This signage may include wording such as 'Stop – Contact precautions required prior to entering room'.

With these types of processes already in place, the implementation phase becomes simple, quick and effective.

To ensure best clinical outcomes when dealing with infection control issues, it is essential that staff are provided with appropriate ongoing supervision and direction from registered staff members. As particular episodes of infection unfold, the direction of interventions will alter to address any changes. Evolving strategies must be clearly and openly communicated to guarantee all staff are following updated guidelines. Supervisors will be able to confirm that workers understand the procedures and that work practices are correct, effective and appropriate to the situation.

Evaluating the effectiveness of implemented procedures

While it is important to identify situations requiring specific infection control procedures, it is equally as important to evaluate their effectiveness. It is of little benefit to follow set procedures if they do not address the issue or fail completely, such as if infection continues to spread. The evaluation process is paramount to ensuring that the procedure or guideline is effective.

In the event that a procedure is not effective, it is necessary to revise its content as required. Sometimes this occurs simply because it has not been evaluated for some time and is considered out of date.

One of the areas for consideration in the evaluation process is determining whether the procedure or guideline is considered best practice, evidence-based and current. Changes in practice are numerous and frequent as new evidence unfolds. Keeping abreast of new developments is a professional obligation and innovations in practice are necessary to compare and evaluate current standards and practices.

The evaluation process not only considers practices that are effective and ineffective, but also requires reference to evidenced-based literature such as journal articles, government guidelines and other prominent bodies of relevance such as WHO. These pertinent documents create a benchmark to work towards and must be considered in the evaluation of any healthcare practice, procedure or guideline.

Contributing to ongoing associated quality improvement measures

Quality improvement is everyone's responsibility and as such all healthcare workers are expected to contribute to continuous quality improvement processes. Depending on the nature of the healthcare facility, this may present in different contexts. Some services may have one dedicated team to address all areas of quality improvement, while other services may choose to have separate but dedicated teams for specific areas of concern.

For example, often there are small teams who are dedicated to infection prevention or management or hazard identification. However, the overall goal for each team often has similarities and are guided by the following principles:

- Analyse the cause of the issue.
- Identify possible trends.
- Isolate specific practices that may enable an increased risk of contributing to the issue.
- Evaluate current practice to address the issue.
- Evaluate current monitoring and surveillance procedures that aim to detect and monitor the issue.
- Plan changes as indicated, guided by evidenced-based research.
- Implement and evaluate changes.
- Educate staff on changes and any identified knowledge or skill deficits regarding the issue.
- Promote and sustain any changes with a continued focus on quality improvement.

In order to deliver effective infection control practices, it is imperative that all levels and streams of staff within the clinical setting have a broad working knowledge of infection control principles. Infection control education of all staff will ensure that these principles are not breached inadvertently. Combining this initial level of education with workplace auditing will identify gaps in knowledge that require addressing and will contribute to the maintenance of a baseline standard or expectation. Further information gathered through the quality improvement process can be identified and integrated into current practices through feedback, education and updated work instructions and guidelines.

TIP BOX

Quality improvement process

Make sure that you have a working knowledge of the quality improvement process in place at your facility. This includes a clear understanding of how you may raise issues that you have identified as requiring improvement.

SUMMARY

- Organisational policies and procedures form the fundamental basis for effective infection control practices.
- Healthcare organisations are obliged to provide comprehensive policies and procedures that are easily accessible to staff.
- Healthcare workers are obliged to accurately implement policies and procedures and acknowledge the link they have to current legislation.
- It is imperative that healthcare workers are acutely aware of circumstances requiring the implementation of specific policies and procedures.

- Infection control policies and procedures, once accessed and understood, must be acted upon.
- Interventions that require prompt application of infection control policies and procedures must be accompanied by an evaluation process.
- It is crucial to acknowledge that these actions contribute to the overall quality improvement in infection control and healthcare practices.

REVIEW QUESTIONS

1 Discuss the importance and goal of staff immunisation policies.
2 Which document would you refer to in order to ascertain your facility's approved method for inserting an indwelling urinary catheter? Where would you expect to find this information?
3 Discuss your understanding of the quality improvement process and your associated role.
4 Discuss the role of the public health unit.
5 A new health worker approaches you for direction regarding emptying a urinary catheter bag. Discuss your response.

7 WASTE MINIMISATION, ENVIRONMENTAL RESPONSIBILITY AND SUSTAINABLE PRACTICE ISSUES

LEARNING OBJECTIVES

At the end of this chapter, you will be able to:

- understand waste minimisation and the implications this has for the environment and issues of sustainability
- identify policy and codes of practice that support environmental sustainability
- recognise the human costs from healthcare-related waste in the context of the healthcare environment.

Introduction

Waste minimisation is not a unique concept to healthcare settings alone. It has become a universal priority for industries and businesses around the world largely due to environmental impacts. The impetus for waste minimisation has other driving factors as well, not least of which include efficiency, economic gain and environmental sustainability. According to the 7th edition of the *Industry Code of Practice for the Management of Biohazardous Waste 2014 (including Clinical & Related Wastes)*, clinical waste relates to any bodily fluids and items contaminated in the same manner that potentially carry and can transmit pathogens.

Healthcare environments have the additional responsibility of ensuring that waste production does not harm those who are exposed to it (**Figure 7.1**). It would be a contradiction for a healthcare setting, whose aim is to promote health and prevent

FIGURE 7.1 Hazardous medical waste

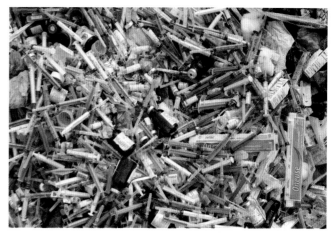

Source: Tim Gainey/Alamy

illness, to cause harm and disease due to poor waste management processes. Therefore, it is imperative that waste minimisation and issues of **sustainability** are everyone's responsibility, especially in a healthcare setting.

Environmental impacts and associated costs of healthcare-related waste

A typical healthcare setting is a large consumer of natural resources including water, energy and requirements for raw materials. This level of consumption and associated waste production has a direct impact on the environment and, consequently, implications for sustainability.

Costs of healthcare-related waste

Although the environmental impact cannot be denied, the other problem with high levels of resource consumption and waste production is the issue of cost.

Healthcare facilities generate huge amounts of waste. The costs associated with the disposal of this waste is directly linked to the type of waste that is being handled. General waste, such as accumulated in private homes, costs the least to dispose of. There are no added handling or transportation considerations to be paid for. This waste would be considered relatively safe to handle. However, clinical, chemotherapeutic or infectious waste poses an increased risk to the environment, as well as those dealing with the disposal of this waste. Extra safeguards must be employed

to minimise the impact on people and the environment. These safeguards cost money, but are essential components to ensuring responsible and safe waste disposal.

For example, the cost of packaging, transporting and incinerating bodily waste from a surgical area such as theatre are approximately twice as much as those associated with the disposal of general waste. Inappropriate disposal of general waste items into clinical, chemotherapeutic or infectious waste receptacles directly inflates overall waste disposal costs. Ensuring correct segregation of waste into appropriate receptacles will translate into significant cost saving for healthcare facilities (Pyrek, 2011).

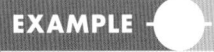

EXAMPLE

Cost of waste removal

The New South Wales (NSW) health sector is responsible for over 200 general hospitals. In 2002, a study was conducted by the Audit Office of New South Wales to analyse the costs incurred for waste removal and disposal. The list below outlines these costs for four hospitals with varying bed capacities:

- Cowra general hospital = $10 306
- Orange general hospital = $95 580
- Concord general hospital = $348 071
- Royal Prince Alfred (RPA) = $755 257

These costs do not include wages apportioned to staff who handle the waste within the hospital.

Environmental impacts of healthcare-related waste

One of the recommendations outlined by the Australian Government Department of Human Services' *Environmental Sustainability Policy* (2014) includes a review of natural resource consumption with an emphasis on the sustainable use of energy. The Australian Government acknowledges that the enormous consumption of energy by healthcare settings has had a detrimental impact on the environment. This includes significant greenhouse gas emissions such as carbon dioxide, methane, nitrous oxide, sulphur hexafluoride, hydrofluorocarbons and perfluorocarbons.

Besides the costly exercise of waste disposal, the method of incineration also presents significant costs to the environment. The emissions include mercury, sulphur dioxide and other toxic by-products that both harm the environment and often end up in our air, waterways and food supplies. Sulphur dioxide is a by-product produced during incineration of medical waste. This toxic substance is a respiratory irritant and is linked to cardiopulmonary diseases including lung cancer (Pyrek, 2011).

Mercury, another by-product produced by medical waste incineration, is converted into methylmercury. Methylmercury particulates are deposited and dissolved in the sediment of waterways. Fish ingest this heavy metal and when they are consumed by people the mercury is introduced into the human food chain.

While there are alternatives to incineration, there is much debate over the efficacy of these practices and if they actually reduce environmental impacts (Climate and Health Alliance, 2013).

According to the World Health Organization, mercury is considered to be 'one of the top ten chemicals or groups of chemicals of major public health concern' (WHO, 2013).

Mercury is a direct threat to the development of unborn children and may have toxic effects on numerous body organs, including lungs, kidneys, skin, eyes, nervous system, digestive system and immune system (WHO, 2013).

Policy and codes of practice supporting environmental sustainability

According to the *Environmental Sustainability Policy* (2014), there are many strategies that healthcare settings can implement to minimise waste production, protect the environment and increase sustainability.

Minimising packaging

One of the first recommendations is to better analyse the procurement of products. This includes placing a sense of social responsibility on manufacturers, including the limitation of packaging. Most packaging consists of plastic-based products that pose a particularly challenging residual problem for the environment. Choosing products that minimise the use of plastics, including in packaging, reduces not only costs but also environmental impacts.

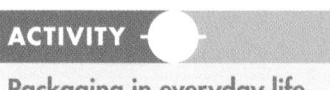

ACTIVITY

Packaging in everyday life
Take a moment to think about the packaging from purchases that you encounter in your day-to-day life.
    Identify three specific examples of situations where the use of packaging could be reduced.

Reviewing consumption of natural resources

The following presents a summary of the *Industry Code of Practice for the Management of Biohazardous Waste (including Clinical & Related Wastes)* (2014) 6th and 7th editions' recommendations for waste minimisation strategies that are being implemented across Australia as best practice guidelines.

Waste minimisation from product procurement

The healthcare industry is responsible for purchasing goods that cause the least harm to the environment, both when products are in use and after use, especially in regard to end-of-life disposal.

Management involvement

Healthcare management have a duty of care to ensure the socially responsible and ethical management of waste handling, disposal and transport in line with current legislation and best practice guidelines.

Waste handling techniques

The handling of waste is given extra attention as this is one of the most vulnerable times for transmission. Staff education is paramount to ensuring procedures are followed. Techniques include correct segregation and labelling, alongside simple measures such as adequate supply of correctly marked bins and ensuring that waste is not double-handled in any way.

Home-based healthcare

Any home-based healthcare waste is to be treated exactly the same as in a facility. Services conducting home healthcare must develop a waste management plan just as a large hospital would.
    Too often, healthcare personnel are transporting waste such as sharps bins in ordinary vehicles and this poses a huge risk for transmission.

Clinical waste treatment and disposal methods

The minimum requirement is that clinical waste must be made non-identifiable and non-infectious. The leftover waste must be either fit for disposal or able to be re-used in some way.

Sampling and microbial testing

Any equipment used in the disposal of waste must comply with sampling standards and have a built-in ability to take random and scheduled tests to establish the environmental footprint that is left after the procedure.

Residual disposal

Untreated clinical waste is no longer accepted as landfill. There are quite stringent criteria and treatment processes in place before general landfill is considered as an option. Even the by-products of waste are highly controlled and regulated. At the completion of waste treatment, if the substance is still deemed hazardous, then it will be transported to a specialised disposal facility.

Occupational risk and assessment

It is imperative that workplace health and safety protocols are closely adhered to in order to avoid accidental injury or disease. Risk assessments are commonplace, as are risk control strategies. In particular, radioactive exposure is a significant risk and therefore all waste facilities must have the means of detecting any radioactive waste that is brought to a site. Equally important is ensuring adequate ventilation and safety equipment for all employees.

Emergency plans

The waste facility has the responsibility of developing emergency plans in line with the Environmental Protection Agency. These include:

- establishing potential emergencies that may occur
- outlining possible scenarios and courses of action
- determining hierarchy and delegation of employees
- developing an emergency signal or siren and designating assembly points in the event of evacuation.

Employee responsibilities and training

Competency-based training is essential as part of induction and also as an ongoing practice. There are specific requirements depending on the nature of the job role, such as a hazardous goods and transport licence, but there are also some general training considerations, such as:

- using personal protective equipment specific to that area
- understanding risk and hazard identification
- understanding risk management concepts
- understanding policies and procedures
- identifying occupational exposure risks
- managing emergencies
- complying with legislative requirements.

Promoting sustainability in healthcare

The issue of sustainability must be looked at holistically. It is not solely the job of cleaning or auxillary staff who handle the bulk of healthcare waste; rather, sustainability must be integrated into all organisational practices by all employees. This requires a shift in organisational culture that can only be fostered by education, leadership, accountability and staff engagement.

One of the obstacles to making this shift is the immense pressure that healthcare professionals are under to 'do more with less and quicker'. However, it has been suggested that healthcare professionals will appreciate the significance of sustainability practices if made aware of the link between health and environment.

About 70 per cent of the health budget is dedicated to chronic disease treatment and ongoing management. Many chronic diseases that currently plague our communities are aggravated by the environment. In particular, the industrialised world has many environmental pollutants that affect the development and maintenance of chronic disease and consequently create a burden on healthcare provision. The following case study illustrates an Australian initiative that aims to mitigate environmental impacts from healthcare services and promote practices and infrastructure embedded with principles of sustainability.

CASE STUDY

'Greening' healthcare facilities

The Green Building Council Australia (GBCA) has created a voluntary environmental rating system that aims to assess and minimise the environmental impacts of building construction and design, including developments in healthcare.

GBCA's Green Star – Healthcare v1 tool provides information and support to guide health services to create facilities that:

- provide better health outcomes for patients and staff alike
- receive formalised acknowledgment of environmentally friendly and sustainable practices
- accrue financial savings.

The Flinders Medical Centre expansion was the first healthcare facility to attain the Green Star certification.

In comparison to a similar facility, the Flinders Medical Centre:

- uses 42 per cent less energy
- saves $400 000 on energy costs
- consumes 20 per cent less water
- has reduced carbon dioxide emissions by 4160 tonnes, the equivalent of removing over 800 cars per year from the road
- reduces greenhouse emissions by 45 per cent by using energy-efficient techniques in regards to heating and cooling as well as lighting
- mostly uses its own rainwater collection and re-uses waste water as appropriate.

Source: Adapted from Green Building Council Australia (2012). *Flinders Medical Centre: New South Wing.* http://www.gbca.org.au/gbc_scripts/js/tiny_mce/plugins/filemanager/Flinders_Medical_Centre__New_South_Wing.pdf

Questions

1 Reflect on the case study and outline one of the most significant strategies that assist in minimising energy use.
2 State one main advantage of using a 'green' approach.
3 In accordance with the Green Star principles, identify one initiative that could be implemented in any of your local healthcare settings.

Sustainability in practice

Yet another initiative that is beginning to evolve within Australia is the composting of hospital food waste and other sustainable practices. The Royal Adelaide Hospital is introducing sustainable practices into many areas of operation, and is achieving admirable results in reducing their carbon footprint and reducing waste management bills (Zero Waste, SA).

Source: Zero Waste SA (2014). *Case study: Upclose: Royal Adelaide Hospital*. Government of South Australia. http://www.zerowaste.sa.gov.au/industry/case-studies /government-and-education/royal-adelaide-hospital-and-zero-waste-sa

The human cost of healthcare-related waste management techniques

For those people who work with healthcare-related waste and those who may live nearby, there are numerous and varied health risks. In particular, emissions from incinerators can cause health hazards to those exposed to the fumes. **Table 7.1** provides a summary of common toxins and consequent health disorders arising from exposure.

TABLE 7.1 Common health related toxins and consequent health disorders

Toxin or risk	Health disorder or damage
Mixed emissions	Cardiovascular and respiratory illnesses
Mercury and cadmium	Compromised immune system, nervous system, respiratory system and kidneys
Dioxins, furans and polycyclic aromatic hydrocarbons	Cancer in various body systems
Incinerator ash (often contains high levels of heavy metals and other toxins)	This can often transform into dioxins and furans, causing the same health concerns as mentioned above
Burnt out needles and glass from medical waste	Sharps injury with possibly dire consequences should an individual contract an infectious disease such as HIV
Chemical contaminants or associated pathogens found in landfill sites when they leach from the original site	Respiratory disorders, skin reactions and digestive disorders
Controlled or even uncontrolled fires on landfill sites	The toxins produced from chemicals burning can cause any of the disorders already mentioned

The World Health Organization (WHO) has made recommendations for waste-related healthcare management based on the report entitled *Safe management of wastes from health-care activities* (Chartier et al., 2014). See **Table 7.2**.

TABLE 7.2 Safe strategies for the management of healthcare related waste

Short-term strategies	Medium-term strategies	Long-term strategies
Ensuring that syringes are all made from the one type of plastic to enable ease of recycling	Reduction in frequency of injections and therefore related waste	Escalation of non-incineration technologies and research for the disposal of healthcare waste to prevent disease and exposure to dioxins and furans
Elimination of polyvinyl chloride (PVC) products as they harm the environment	More research into the occupational and non-occupational exposure to emissions	Better support for countries who are developing a national guidance manual for the effective management of healthcare waste
Enabling better and more uniform recycling programs specifically for healthcare and related waste	Risk assessment comparing occupational exposure to incineration to other healthcare-related wastes	Better support to countries in developing and implementing a national plan, related policies and legislation regarding healthcare waste.
Conduct or contribute to research that considers alternatives to incineration, which poses a huge hazard to the environment and human health		Promotion of environmentally sound principles in healthcare waste management as demonstrated in the Basel Convention
Better waste reduction and segregation practices		Better support including human and financial resources to safely manage healthcare waste in all countries
Better placement of incinerators away from the bulk of people and also better control measures for monitoring the emissions		

The importance of data collection

A Victorian Government initiative (2008) estimated approximately 260 million kilograms of dense waste is generated by our hospitals in Australia. The report stated that it could not quantify how much of that waste could be apportioned to particular hospitals due to lack of data collection in this area.

Increased resources for information gathering and reporting could greatly assist in better waste management practices.

This is now of great significance as healthcare services continue to expand at five per cent per year and therefore related waste also increases.

Source: Department of Human Services (2008). *Waste minimisation in healthcare: User guide*. Victorian Government. http://docs.health.vic.gov.au /docs/doc/818B9B462215777FCA25798100819C6B/$FILE /waste-minimisation.pdf

The need for further research

Finally, there is an urgent need for further research and development regarding the health consequences experienced by people who work with healthcare-related waste or are exposed to it in any way. To date, there is only a small body of research that reports on the risks and related effects of healthcare-related waste exposure.

By investing in this type of research, healthcare providers are better placed to plan, implement and evaluate preventative and protective strategies. Not least of all, the environmental impacts should also factor into this planning process.

Overall, waste minimisation strategies can be seen to have a three-fold knock on effect:

1 Reduction in environmental damage
2 Reduction in health-related disorders and diseases
3 Significant financial savings, hopefully meaning that the healthcare dollar can be stretched further than previously anticipated

SUMMARY

- Waste minimisation in a healthcare setting is directly linked to increased sustainability of service delivery. It is everyone's responsibility and as such all employees can make valuable contributions
- Healthcare facilities are becoming much more conscious of waste minimisation and its link to environmental impacts, cost and sustainability. Policies and codes of practice are being developed to support this direction. Students and staff need to be aware of these policies and practices to assist in supporting effective implementation.
- Students and staff should be aware that by assisting to reduce healthcare-related waste, there will be an associated reduction in disease and an increase of available funds that can be more effectively used in other areas of the healthcare environment.

REVIEW QUESTIONS

1 Most healthcare settings are large consumers of resources. List three resources that are required for the safe and efficient running of a healthcare facility.
2 State one waste disposal method that causes harmful emissions that have a direct impact on the environment and people's health.
3 Discuss one social responsibility that healthcare providers are accountable for when purchasing goods.
4 Define clinical waste.
5 In regards to clinical waste management, what is one of the most vulnerable times for transmission of infection.
6 State three employee responsibilities in relation to waste management.
7 Discuss two recent innovations in waste minimisation management.
8 Within an acute healthcare setting, name the department that is responsible for the majority of waste production.
9 State one benefit of Green Star ratings for clinical settings.
10 Discuss one short-term strategy for safer waste management in accordance with WHO recommendations.

APPENDIX A: AUSTRALIAN, STATE AND TERRITORY LEGISLATIVE REQUIREMENTS

Overarching Commonwealth laws, also referred to as Acts, detail health and safety concepts, among others, that are directly related to infection control and safe practise. Regulations are a set of mandatory requirements that comply with an Act. Every State and Territory of Australia has its own interpretation of the Act, and thus its own Regulations. The local health and safety authority then administers those regulations, hence why the laws vary across the country.

The following table lists the relevant legislation and standards in Australia, inclusive of States and Territories, that pertain to infection control within the healthcare environment.

	Standards and legislation	Topics covered
Australia	*Work Health and Safety Act 2011*	
ACT	**Work Health and Safety Regulation 2011 SL2011-36** **Republication number 17, effective from 21 May 2015** Administered by Work Safe Australian Capital Territory (www.worksafe.act.gov.au)	• Workplace health and safety • Standard and transmission-based precautions, including the use of PPE • Safe handling use and disposal of sharps • Reprocessing of re-usable medical equipment, including the act of disinfection and sterilisation
QLD	**Work Health and Safety Regulation 2011** **Effective from 24 October 2014** Administered by Workplace Health and Safety Queensland (https://www.worksafe.qld.gov.au/)	
NSW	**Work Health and Safety Regulation 2011** **Effective from 4 June 2015** Administered by the Work-Cover Authority of New South Wales (www.workcover.nsw.gov.au)	
TAS	**Work Health and Safety Regulation 2012** Administered by Workplace Standards Tasmania (www.wst.tas.gov.au)	
SA	**Work Health and Safety Regulations 2012** Administered by SafeWork SA	

	Standards and legislation	Topics covered
VIC	Occupational Health and Safety Regulations 2007 is made under the *Occupational Health and Safety Act 2004* Administered by WorkSafe Victoria (www.worksafe.vic.gov.au)	
WA	Occupational Safety and Health Regulations 1996 is made under the *Occupational Safety and Health Act 1984* Administered by WorkSafe Western Australia (www.safetyline.wa.gov.au)	
Australia and New Zealand	Australia/New Zealand. Standard, AS/NZS 4187: 2003 Cleaning, disinfecting and sterilizing reusable medical and surgical instruments and equipment, and maintenance of associated environments in healthcare facilities	• Cleaning
Australia and New Zealand	AS/NZS 4031:1992 Non-reusable containers for the collection of sharp medical items used in healthcare areas	• Sharps containers
Australia and New Zealand	AS/NZS 4261:1994 Reusable containers for the collection of sharp items used in human and animal medical applications	

APPENDIX B: INFECTION CONTROL ORIENTATION

Handwashing assessment

At the start of employment, you are expected to competently *demonstrate* a social handwash. During the orientation stage you may be asked to perform this task as evidence of your competence.

Similarly, it is expected that you would have existing *knowledge* regarding hand hygiene. This includes the significance of the '5 Moments for Hand Hygiene'. Most facilities now align themselves with the WHO Multimodal Hand Hygiene Improvement Strategy.

Take a moment to recall the '5 Moments for Hand Hygiene'. As part of this infection control orientation, please visit http://www.hha.org.au/ > Online learning packages.

Complete the online learning package that is relevant to your discipline area; for example, nursing, medical, allied health. Remember to email a copy of your certificate to your manager on completion and also keep a copy for your own records. It is standard practice to conduct this online learning package on an annual basis.

WHO handwashing questionnaire for healthcare workers

As part of your infection control orientation, please complete the 'Hand Hygiene Knowledge Questionnaire'. It can be found at http://www.who.int/ > Programmes > Clean care is safer care > Save lives and clean your hands > Tools and resources > Evaluation and feedback. Choose the 'Hand Hygiene Knowledge Questionnaire for Health-Care Workers'.

Save lives: clean your hands video

For a powerful reminder of how hand hygiene can touch individual lives, visit http://www.who.int/ > Programmes > Clean care is safer care > Save lives and clean your hands and on the right side of the page choose 'Hand hygiene related videos and podcasts'. Click on the title *Save lives: clean your hands*.

Perception survey for healthcare workers

In order to consolidate this information, it is worthwhile taking the time to complete another questionnaire created by WHO. This aims to capture a sense of the healthcare worker's perceptions and behaviours relating to hand hygiene as well as test their knowledge.

To complete this survey, visit http://www.who.int/ > Programmes > Clean care is safer care > Save lives and clean your hands > Tools and resources > Evaluation and feedback. Click on *Perception Survey for Health-Care Workers*.

Waste management

The following information highlights the importance of waste management strategies and provides a working knowledge of standard procedures within most healthcare environments.

Sharps

To gain an understanding of your facility's sharps disposal guidelines, read the policies and procedures relating to sharps and answer the following questions:

1   Other than used needles and syringes, what else must be disposed of in a sharps container? For example, do used razors and blood sugar lancets get disposed of in a sharps bin in accordance with facility policy or is there an alternative?
2   Are sharps bins located in every room or at certain central locations?
3   Locate all of the sharps bins in the facility.
4   How do you dispose of full sharps bins?
5   Where are the new sharps bins stored?

Clinical waste

It is important to gain the knowledge of clinical waste management pertaining to your facility. Read any policies or procedures relating to clinical waste management and answer the following questions:

1   What is the definition of clinical waste in your facility?
2   What are the handling expectations, such as the use of gloves?
3   What are the disposal expectations (double bagging and specialised/colour-coded rubbish bags)?
4   Locate all of the clinical waste bins in the facility.
5   Who is responsible for emptying these bins and how often is this completed?
6   Are there any special arrangements for disposal during times of reduced staffing such as on public holidays?

General waste

It is also vital to understand the difference between clinical waste and general waste, as the facility will have differing management protocols for each. Read any policies or procedures relating to general waste and answer the following questions:

1   What is the definition of general waste in your facility?
2   What are the handling expectations, such as the use of gloves?
3   What are the disposal expectations; for example, do general waste bins need to have a lid or specialised structure?
4   Locate all of the general waste bins in your facility.
5   Who is responsible for emptying these bins and how often is it completed?
6   Are there any special arrangements for disposal during times of reduced staffing such as public holidays?

Linen management

As a healthcare worker it is also important to understand the facility's procedures when handling and managing linen. Read any policies, procedures or protocols relating to linen management and answer the following questions:

1   Which linen is laundered by an outside contractor?
2   Which linen is washed on site?
3   Are patients/residents expected to wash any of their own linen or clothing? What does this entail?
4   How is contaminated linen managed (e.g. a sheet that has become heavily contaminated by faeces)?

5 Are there any specialised bags, which disintegrate during the cleaning process, available for contaminated items to be placed in prior to washing?

Use of PPE

While you are expected to understand the use of PPE, take time during orientation to read the facility's policies and procedures relating to this topic and answer the following questions:

1 In accordance with your facility's guidelines, what is PPE?
2 Identify three tasks within your role where you would need to use PPE and list the items required.
3 Where are each of these items kept in your facility?
4 How are stocks of these items replenished and where are they stored?
5 To whom and how would you report if a PPE item was missing or faulty?

Precautions: Droplet, contact and airborne

Part of your infection control orientation is to identify your facility's policies and procedures regarding additional precautions. After reading these documents you will need to answer the following questions:

1 In accordance with your facility's policies, what are droplet, contact and airborne precautions and when are they implemented?
2 Who can initiate the implementation of these precautions?
3 Where would you find the necessary PPE to implement these precautions?

4 Where is signage regarding these precautions kept and where should it be placed once these steps have been implemented?
5 How are stock and PPE items replaced after the precautions cease?
6 Does your facility conduct a 'terminal' clean at the end of an isolation case and what does this involve (e.g. are curtains laundered)?

Antimicrobial stewardship

Does your facility have a statement regarding antimicrobial stewardship? In the event that your facility has not yet developed a statement on antimicrobial stewardship, liaise with your superiors to establish what work has been undertaken towards its development and ask if there any tasks that you could conduct to contribute to its development. Alternatively, conduct your own research regarding antimicrobial stewardship and feed the information back to management and, with permission, also to the rest of the healthcare team at your facility. You will need to use the questions below as a guide to your research.

If you have located your facility's antimicrobial stewardship statement, read the document and answer the following questions:

1 What is the definition of antimicrobial stewardship?
2 What is antimicrobial resistance?
3 How has this resistance proliferated?
4 Outline one strategy that will improve the appropriateness of antimicrobial use.
5 State one annual campaign that aims to raise awareness of antimicrobial stewardship.

6 Describe one simple educational activity that could be or has been conducted in relation to antimicrobial stewardship.

Isolation

Study the available policies, procedures and resources in your facility regarding the use of isolation and answer the following questions:

1 In accordance with facility guidelines, under what circumstances is the isolation of patients/residents commenced?

2 Provide an example of an infection that would require isolation due to the implementation of:

a droplet precautions

b airborne precautions

c contact precautions.

3 Where is your facility's isolation kit/s located?

4 Perform an audit of the contents of the isolation kit (as guided by the inventory attached to the kit) to identify if any items are missing.

5 Report back to your superiors on the outcome of the audit and ensure items are replaced if required.

Staff health status

The role of a healthcare worker also means taking the necessary steps to protect one's own health and safety. This includes ensuring that all clinically indicated immunisations are current and staff have an understanding of the risks associated with exposure prone procedures and the identification of workplace hazards. Please refer to your policies and procedures documents regarding these issues to have a better understanding of how they relate to the context of your workplace.

Immunisations

As part of your orientation period, ensure that you have supplied evidence of the following immunisations:

- MMR (measles, mumps, rubella)
- Hepatitis B
- Varicella (chicken pox)
- DTP (diphtheria, tetanus and pertussis)

There are other vaccinations that may be required when working in speciality areas such as with Aboriginal and Torres Strait Islander people and in neonate units. The list above is a generic list and other immunisations can be added. Check with your employer which immunisations are required.

Exposure prone procedures

Within your facility, locate and read the policies and procedures pertaining to exposure prone procedures and answer the following questions:

1 What is an exposure prone procedure?

2 Provide an example where you may be involved in an exposure prone procedure.

3 In accordance with your facility's policy, what would you do if you experienced a needle stick injury?

4. Who do you report a needle stick injury to and what paperwork would be required for completion of the incident?
5. Where would you find this paperwork?
6. What follow up is required after a needle stick injury?

Occupational hazards

Locate and read any policies, procedures or protocols about occupational hazards within your facility. Answer the following questions:

1. What is an occupational hazard?
2. What would you do if you identified a hazard in your workplace?
3. After completing a tour of your facility, try to find a potential or actual workplace hazard.
4. On identifying a workplace hazard, who would you inform and what paperwork would need to be completed?
5. Where is this paperwork located?

APPENDIX C: OUTBREAK MANAGEMENT

Outbreak management checklist

Action	Completed
Is there an outbreak?	
• Are there two or more cases of suspected infection?	☐
• Has a source of outbreak been identified?	☐
Has the outbreak management team been notified?	☐
Have staff been notified?	☐
All staff involved in providing services within the suspected outbreak area must be notified and plans implemented to restrict staff movement through the area to decrease risk of spread. This includes:	☐
• medical officers	☐
• clerical staff	☐
• operational support officers	☐
• cleaning staff	☐
• allied health professionals	☐
• pharmacy staff	☐
• volunteers	☐
• delivery staff	☐
Have visitors and patients been notified?	☐

Action	Completed
Has the type of infection and mode of transmission been identified?	☐
• Allow for provision of appropriate PPE as relevant to mode of transmission.	
Have outbreak kits been distributed and implementation of infection control measures commenced?	
• Have sufficient PPE been provided, such as aprons, gowns, gloves, masks and eyewear?	☐
• Has appropriate hand hygiene measures been reinforced?	☐
• Has appropriate signage been displayed, such as 'Additional Precautions Required'?	☐
• Have affected patients been isolated?	☐
• Have waste disposal receptacles been provided within the patients' room?	☐
Has the facility taken steps to limit spread of infection?	
• Staff appointed to work with affected patients.	☐
• Group patients with the same infection.	☐
• Ensure movement of affected patients is restricted to vital purposes only.	☐
• Restrict visitors, especially highly susceptible hosts.	☐
• Increase frequency and appropriate method of cleaning in affected areas.	☐
Specimen collection	☐
• Has the pathology service been notified of increased specimen collection required?	☐
Has outbreak documentation commenced?	☐
• List all affected patients and staff.	
• Include for each affected person details of symptoms, date of onset and pathology confirmation of disease.	
The running tally of data must be updated at least daily and may require twice daily updating.	

Action	Completed
Have relevant authorities been notified?	☐
• Public Health Unit notified: date: __/__/__	
• Communicable Disease Unit notified: date: __/__/__	
Have reviews been organised?	☐
• These can be daily or twice daily running review.	
Overview report	
• Collation and analysis of data.	☐
• Facility specific plan updated including improvements identified during outbreak.	☐

Outbreak kit suggested contents

It can be very useful to include a suite of documents for facility use within the outbreak kit, in case of an outbreak.

Outbreak kits should be checked regularly to ensure all stock is present and in date.

Signage

- Signage directing visitors to seek information before entering the patients' room
- Signage relevant to mode of transmission of infection

Adequate supply of PPE

- Gowns
- Gloves
- Masks
- Aprons
- Protective eyewear
- Liquid soap
- Alcohol-based hand rub or gel
- Paper towel

Specimen collection items

- Disposable toilet pans
- 'In toilet' specimen collection containers
- Faecal specimen containers
- Labels
- Waterproof, sealable, pathology bags
- Pathology request forms
- Disposable spatulas

Cleaning products and associated equipment

- Bleach and applicator bottle – check expiry date of bleach
- Neutral detergent
- Single use cloths
- Paper towels
- Infectious waste bags
- Linen bags
- Alcohol wipes (minimum 70%)

Staff involvement and roles

When challenged with an outbreak of a communicable disease in a healthcare setting, it is imperative to involve key staff members from each operational area on the Outbreak Management Team. In doing so, all areas of the health service are represented for input and clear staff feedback and direction. The list and associated roles below should be considered dynamic and fluid dependent on the type and size of the organisation. For example, a small residential aged care facility would neither have nor require the same representation as a large metropolitan hospital.

Work stream	Representative	Role in Outbreak Management Team
Hospital executive	CEO or other delegated officer	Oversees process and ensures allocation of required funds
Nominated media officer	Public relations personnel	Delivers information to the media as required following collaborative report formulation
Nursing	Infection control RN Nurse unit managers Clinical nurses Nurse educators	Implementation of all transmission-based precautions as appropriate (e.g. airborne, droplet or contact)
Medical	Emergency department Ward medical officers Pathology staff	Screening of possible outbreak symptoms and making the public aware
Food services	Chefs Meal delivery and collection services	The implementation of disposable eating utensils and extra food handling precautions as required Limit or eliminate contact with infectious patients

Work stream	Representative	Role in Outbreak Management Team
Operational services officers	Cleaning services Laundry/linen management Bed cleaners Linen transportation Pathology deliveries Operating theatre assistants Porterage Environmental officers	Additional cleaning requirements such as 'terminal' cleans of patient rooms on clearance Ensuring that extra waste disposal services are implemented as required Ensure essential business continues with infection control adjustments as necessary limiting or eliminating any contact with infectious patients
Security services	Security officers	Limit or eliminate contact with infectious patients
Pharmacy	Pharmacist	Limit or eliminate contact with infectious patients
Clerical/office staff	Receptionist Administration staff	Limit or eliminate contact with infectious patients
Diversional therapy/lifestyle officers	Physiotherapists	Limit or eliminate contact with infectious patients
Maintenance	Maintenance staff Cleaners	Limit or eliminate contact with infectious patients
Volunteers	Regular 'in house' volunteer workers	Limit or eliminate contact with infectious patients

It is imperative that managers and key stakeholders communicate clearly with other stakeholders and external contractors to ensure that these people are not exposed to any infectious agents and that transmission to others and the wider community is eliminated. These stakeholders and contractors may include:

- trades people
- community visitors/justice department
- allied health professionals
- postal service/deliveries
- visitors and family members.

GLOSSARY

access relates to how easy or difficult it is for a person to obtain healthcare services and/or advice

aerobic an organism that must have oxygen in order to survive and grow

airborne carried through the air

airborne precautions guidelines used for patients who are known to be infected and have the possibility of infection transmission via the airborne route

alcohol-based hand rub (ABHR) alcohol-based preparation that is rubbed onto hands with the view of reducing microorganisms and does not require the use of running water as it evaporates

allied health worker (AHW) physiotherapists, occupational therapists, speech pathologists, social workers, podiatrists and their assistants

amoebae a single-celled protozoa that utilises pseudopods to move (eukaryotic organism)

anaerobic an organism that must not have oxygen in order to survive and grow

antibiotic a group of medications that are often used to treat bacterial infections

antibodies a protein produced by the body in response to infection; they are found in the blood and other body fluids; the immunoglobulins are produced by lymphocytes in response to bacteria, viruses and other infections

assistant in nursing (AIN) a worker who has undertaken Certificate III level studies in an area of healthcare, such as aged care; some healthcare providers no longer offer assistant-in-nursing positions, preferring to employ people as personal care workers

asymptomatic without symptoms

bacteria a microorganism that may be capable of causing disease (prokaryotic organism)

bacterial spores *see* endospores

bloodborne viruses (BBVs) viruses that are present in a person's blood and can be transmitted through direct contact with the infected person's blood or bodily fluids; they include HIV, hepatitis B and hepatitis C

bronchoscope an instrument used to examine the bronchus, the large airways of the lungs

candidiasis an overgrowth of *Candida albicans* causing a fungal condition

carrier a person who carries a pathogen with or without symptoms of disease

central line an intravenous line or catheter that is inserted into a large vein (such as the superior vena cava) typically in the neck, to rest near the heart

chemotherapeutic the effect of chemicals that have a toxic effect on microorganisms causing disease or that selectively destroy tumour tissues

chemotherapy refers to the use of any drug to treat disease; however, it is usually used to describe drug therapy used to treat cancer

cholera an acute infectious disease of the small intestine caused by the *Vibrio cholerae* bacillus

CHRISP Centre for Healthcare Related Infection Surveillance and Prevention

ciliates single-celled microorganisms that have multiple cilia (hair-like structures) that propel the cell

clinical handwash a handwash that is conducted prior to performing an invasive procedure and lasts for a minimum of one minute

colonisation the process of microorganisms living and reproducing on the human body without causing disease

congenital existing at or before birth

contact (direct) the transmission of a pathogen from one host to another via physical contact

contact (indirect) the transmission of a pathogen from one host to another via another object

contamination the unwanted presence of microorganisms

cultural awareness having an understanding of other people's backgrounds including country of birth, language, values, customs and beliefs

cultural diversity openly accepting and appreciating the varying backgrounds of people including language, values, customs and beliefs

cultural safety promoting an environment where it is safe for individuals/groups to fully express and embrace their cultural identity

culturally competent healthcare behaviours demonstrated by healthcare workers that indicate a level of proficiency in providing care to clients where their cultural needs, such as language, customs and beliefs, are valued and upheld

cytoplasm the contents of a cell within the membrane except the nucleus

cytotoxic toxic to cells

diabetes the group of diseases characterised by the body not making enough insulin or where the insulin produced is not working

disease a damaging change in either the physiologic or metabolic status of a host

disinfect the destruction of microorganisms, including those that are pathogens, via either physical or chemical processes

DNA deoxyribonucleic acid; the structure that holds genetic information

dormant inactive

droplet transmission the spread of microorganisms through the air in small liquid droplet form

endogenous infection an infection caused by the microorganisms living on the patient's body

endoscope an instrument used to examine the digestive tract by passing the scope down the patient's mouth

endospores a thick-coated structure produced within some bacteria (Gram positive bacteria)

endotracheal tube a flexible cannula introduced orally into the trachea to facilitate a safe airway

enrolled nurse (EN) a nurse who has undertaken Diploma-level studies

equity fairness; relates to whether all people are equally able to access the types of healthcare services required and how these services are distributed

Escherichia coli also known as *E. coli*, a bacteria that normally lives in the intestines of people and animals

eukaryotic an organism that has DNA in a nucleus and also has organelles

exogenous infection an infection caused by microorganisms external to the human body

exudate discharge from a wound

fungi organisms that are not capable of photosynthesis (eukaryotic)

genus a level of a classification system, located above species

Gram the surname of the researcher who established the staining method

Gram negative bacteria that do not have a robust cell membrane and stain red

Gram negative pseudomonas bacteria of the genus *Pseudomonas*

Gram positive bacteria that have a robust cell membrane and stain blue

guideline a document that supports decision making and provides advice on best practice

habitat usual living environment

healthcare associated infections (HAI) infections gained from within a healthcare facility/hospital

healthcare worker (HCW) a person who provides direct patient care or has physical contact with a patient/client; includes dentists, medical practitioners, nurses, assistants-in-nursing, personal care workers, allied health workers, wards people, catering staff, healthcare students, emergency personnel (fire, ambulance and volunteer first aid workers); for infection control purposes, this should also include personnel who have contact with patients' blood or body substances such as laboratory staff, biomedical and engineering staff, mortuary technicians, central sterilising supply staff and staff responsible for cleaning, decontaminating and disposing of contaminated materials

helminths worms

hepatitis A an inflammation of the liver typically caused by ingestion of contaminated food or water

herd immunity the principle that people who have immunity to infectious disease will not carry the pathogen, thereby reducing the incidence of that particular disease in the community, and consequently reducing the chance of encounter by susceptible hosts

host the patient or client that microorganisms live in or on

human immunodeficiency virus (HIV) a retrovirus that causes acquired immunodeficiency syndrome (AIDS)

immunocompromised a condition where a person's immune system is compromised, often through disease or treatment processes

immunosuppressant an agent that causes depression of the immune system

implementation standard a document that specifies the minimum actions required to comply with a policy

incubation the span of time between exposure to a pathogen and the emergence of symptoms

indwelling catheter (IDC) a tube inserted into the bladder via the urethra to drain urine out and into a bag

infection growth and multiplication of pathogens in or on the patient

integumentary system an organ of the body consisting of skin, nails, hair and exocrine glands

intravenous line a cannula placed in a vein to facilitate delivery of fluids and medication

isolation containment of either an infectious client and/or an immunocompromised client in a single room or similar area

latent virus a virus that resides within the body in an inactive state

material safety data sheet (MSDS) the specific documentation outlining the storage and safety requirements of chemicals

men's and women's business the clear demarcations of Aboriginal and Torres Strait Islander cultures of what is appropriate and relevant to be addressed by men and what is to be addressed by women; men cannot be present for women's business and vice versa

methicillin-resistant *Staphylococcus aureus* a strain of *Staphylococcus aureus* that is resistant to most commonly prescribed antibiotics

microbiology the study of microorganisms

microorganism an organism that must be viewed under a microscope due to its size

mode of transmission method of transference of microorganisms

morbidity the burden or proportion of illness in a particular demographic caused by a particular disease or condition

morphology the biological study of the form of living things

mortality the rate of death caused by a particular disease or condition

mucous membranes a lubricating membrane lining the internal surfaces of organs (e.g. the digestive system)

multiple sclerosis (MS) a disease of the central nervous system

mycosis a fungal infection

needle stick injury injury caused by being punctured with a needle that may or may not have been used

NHMRC National Health and Medical Research Council

normal flora microorganisms or bacteria found in or on the body on a semi-permanent basis without causing disease

norovirus a virus affecting the gastrointestinal tract causing vomiting and/or diarrhoea; it is easily transmitted via contact with an infected person, their surroundings, food and water

organism a living entity

P2 respirator a particulate filter mask that provides respiratory protection against airborne pathogens

parasite an organism that requires a host to survive

pathogen an organism that causes disease

pathogenesis the origin and development of a disease

percutaneous endoscopic gastrostomy (PEG) a procedure in which a flexible feeding tube is inserted into the stomach through the abdominal wall

personal care worker (PCW) a worker who may or may not possess a Certificate III level studies at time of employment; they may provide services including assistance with activities of daily living (such as hygiene) as well as personal support services, such as ironing, washing personal clothing, cleaning of the client's immediate environment, cooking and provision of meals

personal protective equipment (PPE) equipment used in the workplace to reduce risks of hazards occurring

pertussis otherwise known as whooping cough, caused by the *Bordetella pertussis* bacteria

policy a document that prescribes intent to achieve a desired outcome

polio (poliomyelitis) a highly contagious disease caused by a virus

polypharmacy use of multiple medications

procedure a recommended set of practices usually presented in a sequential manner

prognosis the likely outcome and rate of a disease process from diagnosis to recovery or possible death

prokaryotic an organism that lacks subcellular structures (organelles)

protocol a document containing specific guidelines, expected to be followed in detail

protozoa single-celled organisms (eukaryotic)

radiotherapy the use of high-energy rays, usually X-rays and similar, to treat disease

registered nurse (RN) a nurse who has undertaken Degree-level studies

reservoir a site where microorganisms exist and act as a source for infection; this might include any person, animal, plant or substance in which an infectious agent normally lives and multiplies

residential aged care facility (RACF) a facility that provides 24-hour residential care for aged care patients

resistant bacteria bacteria that have mutated and increased their defences to antibiotic therapy

RNA ribonucleic acid; a nucleic acid which assists in protein production

skin integrity the quality of a person's skin

social determinants the environmental influences such as where people live

and work, and also the distribution of vital resources such healthcare and education

social/routine handwash an everyday handwash that should be performed for 40–60 seconds prior to any patient contact

sorry business in Aboriginal and Torres Strait Islander cultures, this is a lengthy grieving time devoted to loved ones who have passed away; it can take weeks to carry out and all normal activities are postponed during this time

source of infection pool of pathogens from which infection is spread

species a grouping of similar organisms, the second tier in bacterial classification, below genus

sporozoa a type of protozoa which has no mechanism of movement

standard precautions foundation approaches and practices that enable the prevention and control of infection transmission in a healthcare setting; applied to all patients irrespective of their infection status

***Staphylococcus aureus;* staph** a common bacteria; part of normal flora in the body but has potential to cause infection when outside its normal location

sterilisation a process which destroys and removes all microorganisms including viruses and endospores

strain the third tier of bacterial classification, below species

suprapubic catheter a tube that enters the bladder through the abdominal wall to drain urine

surgical handwash the handwash used prior to surgery that aims to eliminate transient microorganisms on hands by scrubbing the skin and cleaning under the nails, usually with an antimicrobial soap

surveillance types of programs that aim to collect various forms of data in relation to the occurrence of disease

susceptible host a person who is vulnerable to disease

sustainability the process of ensuring that a certain balance is maintained

that discourages the reduction of natural resources

symptom measureable or reportable changes experienced by a client resulting from disease

systemic infection an infection that is not localised to a certain area of the body; it is throughout the entire body

toxoplasmosis a disease caused by *Toxoplasma gondii*, contracted by eating raw or undercooked meats

tracheostomy tube a flexible tube inserted percutaneously into the trachea to facilitate a safe airway

transmission the movement of infectious agents from one person to another

transmission-based precautions types of precautions used in addition to standard precautions and implemented when patients are known to have an infection that can be transmitted via airborne, droplet or contact routes

tuberculosis (TB) a bacterial infection that usually affects the lungs and causes a severe respiratory disease that can be transmitted via both airborne and droplet

transmission; TB can be cured with the correct treatment but has not yet been eradicated across the world; however, it is generally well managed within Australia

typhoid an illness caused by *Salmonella typhi* bacteria

ulcerative colitis a disease characterised by inflammation and micro-ulcers in the superficial layers of the large intestine or colon

urinary tract infection an infection of any part of the urinary tract, most often used in reference to a bladder infection

vaccine a preparation containing antigens used to immunise a person against a specific disease

varicella (chickenpox) an illness that is very contagious and caused by the varicella-zoster virus; it usually starts with flu-like symptoms and then progresses on to a rash with small pink blotches that develop into itchy blisters

vector an organism that transmits pathogens from one infected person to another, such as a mosquito

venepuncture the act of piercing the skin and accessing a vein to take blood from a person

virulence the extent to which an organism is able to cause infection

virus an infectious particle that consists of nucleic acid contained within a protein coat; generally not responsive to antibiotic therapy

World Health Organization (WHO) a not-for-profit organization that directs and coordinates health issues and policies within the United Nations System

Workplace Health and Safety Act 2011 a piece of legislation designed to outline the responsibilities of both the employer and employee in order to keep a workplace safe and healthy

REFERENCES

CHAPTER 1

Anthikad, J. & Sumanaswini, P. (2013). *Medical microbiology for nurses (including parasitology)*. Jaypee Brothers Medical Publishers.

Centre for Healthcare Related Infection Surveillance and Prevention & Tuberculosis Control (CHRISP) (2013). *Guideline for Type and Duration of Precautions for Infectious Diseases and Conditions*. Queensland Government. http://www.health.qld.gov.au/chrisp/policy_framework/guide_precautions.pdf

Crisp, J. & Taylor, C. (2008). *Fundamentals of nursing 3e*. Elsevier Australia.

Health Direct Australia (2014). *Worms in humans*. http://www.healthdirect.gov.au/worms

Lee, G. & Bishop, P. 2010 *Microbiology and infection control for health professionals 4e*. Pearson Australia.

National Center for Emerging and Zoonotic Infectious Diseases (2013). *Hendra virus disease*. US Department of Health and Human Services. http://www.cdc.gov/vhf/hendra/resources/Hendra-FactSheet.pdf

National Health and Medical Research Council (NHMRC) (2010). *Australian Guidelines for the Prevention and Control of Infection in Healthcare*. http://www.nhmrc.gov.au/book/html-australian-guidelines-prevention-and-control-infection-healthcare-2010

Queensland Government (2012). *Methicillin resistant Staphylococcus aureus (MRSA) in the community: Information for clinicians*. Queensland Government. http://www.health.qld.gov.au/chrisp/resources/nmMRSA_clinical.pdf

Queensland Health (2011). *Topic: Staphylococcus aureus infections*. Queensland Government. http://access.health.qld.gov.au/hid/InfectionsandParasites/BacterialInfections/staphylococcusAureusInfection_fs.asp

CHAPTER 2

Division of Viral Diseases, National Center for Immunization and Respiratory Diseases (2013). *Norovirus: Overview*. Centers for Disease Control and Prevention. http://www.cdc.gov/norovirus/about/overview.html

National Health and Medical Research Council (NHMRC) (2010). *Australian Guidelines for the Prevention and Control of Infection in Healthcare*. http://www.nhmrc.gov.au/_files_nhmrc/publications/attachments/cd33_infection_control_healthcare_140616.pdf

Queensland Health (2013). *Topic: Tuberculosis TB*. Queensland Government. http://access.health.qld.gov.au/hid/LungandAirwayHealth/InfectionsandParasites/tuberculosisTb_fs.asp

Queensland Health (2014). *Topic: Chickenpox Varicella*. Queensland Government. http://access.health.qld.gov.au/hid/InfectionsandParasites/ViralInfections/chickenpoxVaricella_fs.asp

The Royal Children's Hospital Melbourne (n.d.). *Washup: Modes of transmission*. http://www.rch.org.au/washup/for_health_professionals/Modes_of_Transmission/

CHAPTER 3

Centre for Healthcare Related Infection Surveillance and Prevention (CHRISP) & Tuberculosis Control (2014). *Guideline for the management of occupational exposure to blood and body fluids*. Queensland Health. http://www.health.qld.gov.au/qhpolicy/docs/gdl/qh-gdl-321-8.pdf

Government of Western Australia (2004). *Environmental Protection (Controlled Waste) Regulations 2004*. http://www.wastenet.net.au/Assets/Documents/Content/Information/Environmental-Protection-Controlled-Waste-Regulations-2004.PDF

Government of Western Australia (2007). *Waste Avoidance and Resource Recovery Act 2007*. State Law Publisher. http://www.slp.wa.gov.au/pco/prod/FileStore.nsf/Documents/MRDocument:5824P/$FILE/WstAvoidanceandResourceRecoveryAct2007_00-00-01.pdf?OpenElement

National Health and Medication Research Council (NHMRC) (1999). *National guidelines for waste management in the health industry* (RESCINDED). https://www.nhmrc.gov.au/_files_nhmrc/publications/attachments/eh11.pdf

National Health and Medical Research Council (NHMRC) (2010). *Australian Guidelines for the Prevention and Control of Infection in Healthcare.* http://www.nhmrc.gov.au/_files_nhmrc/publications/attachments/cd33_infection_control_healthcare_140616.pdf

Office of the Queensland Parliamentary Counsel (2008). *Environmental Protection Regulation 2008.* Queensland Government. https://www.legislation.qld.gov.au/LEGISLTN/CURRENT/E/EnvProtR08.pdf

Office of the Queensland Parliamentary Counsel (2014). *Waste Reduction and Recycling Act 2011.* Queensland Government. https://www.legislation.qld.gov.au/LEGISLTN/CURRENT/W/WasteRedRecA11.pdf

World Health Organization (n.d.). *Clean care is safer care: Tools for evaluation and feedback.* http://www.who.int/gpsc/5may/tools/evaluation_feedback/en/

Zero Waste SA (2010). *Resource Efficiency Assistance Program Snapshot: Waste slashed as Anglicare cuts landfill.* Government of South Australia. http://www.zerowaste.sa.gov.au/upload/REAP/Zero%20Waste%20Snapshot%20Anglicare_WEB_2.pdf

CHAPTER 4

Australian Commission on Safety and Quality in Health Care (ACSQHC) (2010). *The OSSIE Toolkit for implementation of the Australian guidelines for the prevention of infection in health care 2010.* http://www.safetyandquality.gov.au/wp-content/uploads/2012/01/OSSIE-Toolkit_WEB.pdf

Centre for Healthcare Related Infection Surveillance and Prevention (CHRISP) & Tuberculosis Control (2013). *Guideline: Hand hygiene.* Queensland Health. http://www.health.qld.gov.au/qhpolicy/docs/gdl/qh-gdl-321-1-1.pdf

Division of the Chief Health Officer (2010). *Scabies: Management in residential care facilities.* Queensland Government. http://www.health.qld.gov.au/ph/documents/cdb/23496.pdf

Hand Hygiene Australia (2015). *5 Moments for hand hygiene.* http://www.hha.org.au/home/5-moments-for-hand-hygiene.aspx; http://www.hha.org.au/UserFiles/file/Manual/HHAManual_2010-11-23.pdf

Hand Hygiene Australia (2015). *Glove use: Gloves.* http://www.hha.org.au/About/GloveUsePolicy.aspx

Hand Hygiene Australia (2015). *Hand care issues.* http://www.hha.org.au/About/ABHRS/abhr-limitations/hand-care-issues.aspx

Hand Hygiene Australia (2015). *Promotion.* http://www.hha.org.au/ForHealthcareWorkers/promotion.aspx

Hand Hygiene Australia (2015). *What is hand hygiene?* http://www.hha.org.au/AboutHandHygiene.aspx

Ministry of Health NSW (2012). *Policy directive: Environmental cleaning policy.* NSW Government. http://www0.health.nsw.gov.au/policies/pd/2012/pd/PD2012_061.pdf

National Center for Emerging and Zoonotic Infectious Diseases (2014). *Guide to infection prevention for outpatient settings: Minimum expectations for safe care.* http://www.cdc.gov/HAI/pdfs/guidelines/Outpatient-Care-Guide-withChecklist.pdf

National Health and Medical Research Council (NHMRC) (2010). *Australian Guidelines for the Prevention and Control of Infection in Healthcare.* http://www.nhmrc.gov.au/_files_nhmrc/publications/attachments/cd33_infection_control_healthcare_140616.pdf

National Health and Medical Research Council (NHMRC) (2013). *Prevention and control of infection in residential and community aged care.* Commonwealth of Australia. https://www.nhmrc.gov.au/_files_nhmrc/publications/attachments/d1034_infection_control_residential_aged_care_140115.pdf

The Royal Children's Hospital Melbourne (n.d.). *Washup: Modes of transmission.* http://www.rch.org.au/washup/for_health_professionals/Modes_of_Transmission/

World Health Organization (2012). *Hand hygiene in outpatient and home-based care and long-term care facilities: A guide to the application of the WHO multimodal hand hygiene improvement strategy and the 'My Five Moments For Hand Hygiene' approach.* http://apps.who.int/iris/bitstream/10665/78060/1/9789241503372_eng.pdf

CHAPTER 5

Australian Human Rights Commission (2011). 'Chapter 4: Cultural safety and security: Tools to address lateral violence'. *Social Justice Report 2011.* https://www.humanrights.gov.au/publications/chapter-4-cultural-safety-and-security-tools-address-lateral-violence-social-justice

Australian Indigenous Health*InfoNet* (2014). *Overview of Australian Indigenous health status, 2013.* http://www.healthinfonet.ecu.edu.au/health-facts/overviews

Department of Health (2014). *Immunisation coverage data.* Australian Government. http://www.health.gov.au/internet/immunise/publishing.nsf/Content/coverage-data.htm

Department of Immigration and Multicultural Affairs (1998). *A good practice guide for culturally responsive Government services.* Commonwealth of Australia. http://www.immi.gov.au/about/charters/_pdf/culturally-diverse/practice.pdf

Ethnic Communities' Council of Victoria Inc. (2006). *Cultural competence: guidelines and protocols.* http://eccv.org.au/library/doc/CulturalCompetenceGuidelinesandProtocols.pdf

Mackenzie, G.A., Carapetis, J.R., Leach, A.J. & Morris, S.M. (2009). 'Pneumococcal vaccination and otitis media in Australian Aboriginal infants: comparison of two birth cohorts before and after introduction of vaccination'. *BMC Pediatrics,* 9(14). http://www.biomedcentral.com/1471-2431/9/14/

NSW Department of Health (2004). *Communicating positively: A guide to appropriate Aboriginal terminology.* http://www.liveandworkhnehealth.com.au/infobooklets_pdf/CommunicatingPositively.pdf

World Health Organization (2008). *Social determinants of health: Key concepts.* http://www.who.int/social_determinants/thecommission/finalreport/key_concepts/en/

CHAPTER 6

Australian Commission on Safety and Quality in Health Care (ACSQHC) (2011). *National safety and quality health service standards.* http://www.safetyandquality.gov.au/wp-content/uploads/2011/09/NSQHS-Standards-Sept-2012.pdf

Clinical Excellence Commission (n.d.). *Clinical practice improvement program training program.* NSW Department of Health. http://www.cec.health.nsw.gov.au/programs/clinical-practice#overview3

Ministry of Health (2005). *Infection control program quality monitoring.* NSW Department of Health. http://www0.health.nsw.gov.au/policies/PD/2005/pdf/PD2005_414.pdf

Queensland Department of Health (2013). *Guideline: Vaccination of health care workers.* Queensland Government. http://www.health.qld.gov.au/qhpolicy/docs/gdl/qh-gdl-321-9.pdf

Queensland Department of Health (2014). *Guideline: Management of patients with Clostridium difficile infection (CDI).* Queensland Government. http://www.health.qld.gov.au/qhpolicy/docs/gdl/qh-gdl-408.pdf

Queensland Department of Health (2014). *Management of vancomycin resistant enterococcus (VRE).* Queensland Government. http://www.health.qld.gov.au/chrisp/resources/vre.asp

Queensland Department of Health (2014). *Work health and safety risk management implementation standard.* Queensland Government. http://www.health.qld.gov.au/qhpolicy/docs/imp/qh-imp-401-3.pdf

CHAPTER 7

ale.livs (avatar) (2013). *New WHO Handbook on healthcare waste management.* Health Care Without Harm. https://noharm-global.org/articles/news/global/new-who-handbook-healthcare-waste-management

Biohazard Waste Industry (2010). *Industry Code of Practice for the Management of Clinical and Related Wastes, 6th ed.* Waste Management Association of Australia Ltd. http://www.epa.sa.gov.au/xstd_files/Waste/Code%20of%20practice/Code%20of%20Practice%206th%20Edition.pdf

Biohazard Waste Industry (2014). *Industry Code of Practice for the Management of Clinical and Related Wastes,* 7th ed. Waste Management Association of Australia Ltd.

Chartier, Y., Emmanuel, J., Pieper, U., Pruss, A., Rushbrook, P., Stringer, R., Townend, W., Wilburn, S. and Zghondi, R. (Eds) (2014). *Safe management of wastes from health-care activities.* 2nd edition. World Health Organization. http://www.who.int/water _sanitation_health/medicalwaste/wastemanag /en/

Department of Housing and Public Works (Qld) (2014). *Procurement guidance: Integrating sustainability into the procurement process.* Queensland Government. http://www .hpw.qld.gov.au/sitecollectiondocuments /procurementguideintegratingsustainability.pdf

Department of Human Services (2014). *Environmental sustainability policy.* Australian Government. http://www.humanservices.gov .au/corporate/publications-and-resources /environmental-policy

Department of Human Services (VIC) (2008). *Waste minimisation in healthcare: User guide.* Victorian Government. http://docs. health.vic.gov.au/docs/doc/818B9B462215

777FCA25798100819C6B/$FILE /waste-minimisation.pdf

Green Building Council Australia (2011). *Flinders Medical Centre – New South Wing.* http:// www.gbca.org.au/gbc_scripts/js/tiny_mce /plugins/tilemanager/Flinders_Medical_Centre __New_South_Wing.pdf

Harris, N., Pisa, L., Talioaga, S. & Vezeau, T. (2009). 'Hospitals going green: A holistic view of the issue and the critical role of the nurse leader'. Lippincott Nursing Center. http:// www.nursingcenter.com/lnc/pdfjournal ?AID=848644&an=00004650-200903000 -00007&Journal_ID=&Issue_ID=

Lillis, K. (2014). '*Washable keyboards helps hospitals tackle cross contamination'. Infection Control Today.* http://www. infectioncontroltoday.com/~/media /Files/Medical/Whitepapers/2014/05 /washable-keyboards.ashx

National Health and Medical Research Council (NHMRC) (2010). *Australian Guidelines for the Prevention and Control of Infection in Healthcare.* http://www.nhmrc.gov.au/ _files_nhmrc/publications/attachments/cd33 _infection_control_healthcare_140616.pdf

Pyrek, K.M. (2011). Achieving Healthcare Sustainability: Suggestions for Success. *Infection Control Today.* http://www.infectioncontroltoday .com/articles/2011/11/achieving-healthcare -sustainability-suggestions-for-success.aspx

Sunshine Coast Council (QLD) (n.d.). *Sustainable waste management fact sheet.* http://www .sunshinecoast.qld.gov.au/addfiles/documents /waste/sustainable_waste_mgmt.pdf

The Audit Office of New South Wales (2002). *Auditor-General's Report: Performance Audit: Managing hospital waste.* https://www.audit .nsw.gov.au/AOReportSearch.aspx?yBase=3& yrf=2001&yrt=2003&ids=35,&pageModule= 465&ModuleID=821 > Managing Hospital Waste - 2002 Reports

World Health Organization (2013). *Media centre: Mercury and health.* http://www.who .int/mediacentre/factsheets/fs361/en/

INDEX